Study planning
- a guidebook for clinical research

Jacob Rosenberg, MD, DSc, FACS

Copyright © 2018 by Jacob Rosenberg

All rights reserved.

No part of this book may be reproduced, distributed, or transmitted in any form or by any means, including photocopying, recording, or other electronic or mechanical methods, without the prior written permission of the author, except in the case of brief quotations embodied in articles or reviews.

ISBN-13: 978-1986696166
ISBN-10: 1986696162

Disclaimer

The information in this book is not intended as a substitute for the medical or legal advice of a trained person.

Although the author has made every effort to ensure that the information in this book was correct at publication time, the author does not assume and hereby disclaim any liability to any party for any loss, damage, or lack of results associated with comments/text made by the author. This book is not intended as a substitute for the legal or medical advice of lawyers or physicians.

Any information in this book should not be deemed as legal or medical advice. The information in this book is best used to supplement your knowledge.

Study planning
a guidebook for clinical research

ULTIMATE RESEARCHER'S GUIDE SERIES
VOLUME 3

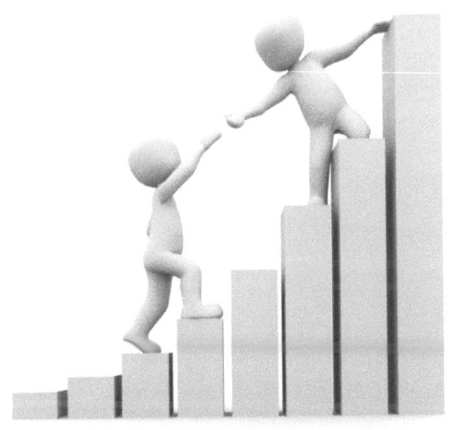

Table of contents

Preface	8
Introduction	12
Chapter 1: Before you start	17
Find a mentor	18
How to get the idea for a project	26
Start writing a systematic review	31
Funding	41
Prepare for the critical phases	51
Chapter 2: Initial study planning	62
Literature search	63
Choose the best study design	79
Feasibility	84
Good Clinical Practice	89
Chapter 3: Now it is getting serious	96
The research protocol	97
The statistical analysis plan	104
The authorship contract	110
Other contracts	119
Permissions and registrations	122
Trial registration	128
Reporting guidelines	134
Chapter 4: Last minute preparations	137
Practical data management	138
Why run a mock patient	141
Who is going to help you	142

Last minute activity	143
Chapter 5: closing	145
closing remarks	146
Other books in this series	148
About the author	150
Notes	152
Contact information	153

Preface

This is the third in a series of books where I will guide you through the different parts of the scientific process in order to improve the overall quality of your research project and thereby hopefully making it easier for you to get your scientific article published in a biomedical journal. The present book is called "study planning" and it will cover the time period from before you start your research career until you are ready to include the first patient in a clinical trial.

The book will have four essential parts being: 1) Before you start 2) Initial study planning 3) Now it is getting serious, and 4) Last minute preparations.

In Part 1 I will discuss how to find a good mentor and how to get the idea for a research project. I will also try to convince you to start your research career by writing a systematic review because it will give you an overview of your research field and at the same time it will also qualify you to probably obtain funding for your research, because now you have already published within the specific field that you will continue your studies within. In Part 1 I will therefore also discuss with you various issues regarding research funding and finally it is important to be aware of possible critical phases that you will meet during your research period, and if you are prepared for that it will of course be easier to survive.

In Part 2 I will discuss the initial study planning including how to search for relevant literature, how to choose the best study design for your research question and discuss why it is very important to look at feasibility before you continue with your planned research. Finally, in Part 2, I will discuss the various regulations including the so-called "Good Clinical Practice" regulations which are in effect by law in Europe. In other parts of the world the rules are essentially the same but they may be called differently.

In Part 3 it is getting a little more serious because now we have to produce a formal research protocol, you have to write a statistical analysis plan and I strongly recommend that you also produce a formal authorship contract already at this point in order not to have problems later on. There may be other contracts that you have to produce and various permissions and registrations that also have to be in place.

In Part 4 I will look at the last preparations that you have to make before you actually include the first patient. This includes how to plan your practical data management because in this area there are quite a lot of things to think about in advance. It is also highly recommendable to run a mock (also called a "pilot") patient before you include the first real patient in your research project because this will show you where you may have some weak spots that can be optimised before you start the real research project.

I hope that the text and discussions in this book will help you to become better prepared before you include your first patient in the research project because needless to say that preparations are extremely important in biomedical research.

The pitfall here, however, may be that you only do preparations and never actually get to the point where you can include a patient in your trial. It is therefore important to plan the preparations and follow a kind of template that you will hopefully find by reading this book. In this way you can prepare efficiently and reasonably fast to continue with patient accrual.

There are undoubtedly many issues regarding study planning that I have not covered in this book so if you have a specific wish for something for future new editions or for another book regarding biomedical research and publishing, then you are more than welcome to write to me. Please use the contact form at the home-page www.biomedicalpublishing.com and I will do my very best to include your ideas in a future book release.

Enjoy!

Introduction

I guess that you have decided to do a clinical trial, and now you are a big question mark and maybe you have worries about the obstacles on your way to being able to start your clinical trial. If you have done it numerous times in the past, then this book may not be for you, but if you are fairly new to clinical research then you will probably find good information in this book.

Nowadays it is absolutely impossible to perform a clinical trial without help. You are not able to do it alone and first of all you need guidance from an experienced person – a so called scientific mentor.

You will often have to find a mentor yourself and in this process the mentor of course has to have experience with clinical research but perhaps more importantly the chemistry between you and your mentor has to be good. You will spend quite a lot of time together and it is important that you can do this without being negative and without struggle.

You may already have a good idea for a

project but I strongly advise that you discuss the idea thoroughly with your scientific mentor as well as with other colleagues before you move on. You also have to read scientific articles within your coming field of research in order to find out if it has already been studied in detail or if there are lacunas that can be covered by you in your upcoming research project.

When you are searching and reading the literature you might as well write a formal systematic review about the research question – why not? You are spending a lot of time searching literature and reading the scientific papers, so why not get something more out of it meaning why not write a good systematic review about the research question. It will be helpful both for readers but also for you personally. You will get a good overview of the research field and at the same time it will also give you a publication on your curriculum vitae which will be important when you are applying for research funding for your project.

There are also mental preparations before you decide to move in to the field of clinical research because you will for sure experience problems along the way and that is why you have to think it through. I certainly do not mean that you should stay away from clinical research, but if you prepare mentally for the critical phases, then it will be much easier for you to go through them and get your study done.

There are, depending on your country, various rules and regulations that you have to comply with but all around the World you will have to obtain permission from a local ethical committee or institutional review board before you can start patient accrual for your study. Depending on the study design and whether you are evaluating drugs or devices there are many other potential registrations and permissions that you have to obtain.

It is important to spend time on good planning. This will include a formal research protocol with a statistical analysis plan and I strongly advise that you also produce an authorship contract so that authorship on the resulting paper(s) will be decided already before you start your study.

You do not have to be a computer genius in order to perform clinical research but you have to think about the practical data management already before you start. Most researchers use simple programs like Excel or a statistical software package, but there are rules about how you should keep your data secured depending on the anonymity of the patients. In the study planning you also have to consider getting practical help because it will be almost impossible for you if you have to obtain all the necessary data for your study without help from other people. Depending on your local organisation it may involve research nurses, medical students or other people that can give you a hand along the way. Do not start your study without some kind of practical help because then you will probably not get through it. Clinical research may be quite hard work and you also have to do other things I presume. So get help.

The entire research process involves study planning, data management including data analysis, knowledge about medical statistics, the entire process of writing the scientific articles and knowledge about biomedical publishing. When you have written your paper and submitted it to a journal you most often have to present it either locally or at national and international congresses or conferences. You will also as a medical researcher need to know about poster-presentations as well as oral presentations. Thus, the research process involves numerous steps. The present book will cover various issues of study planning and the other books in this book series will try to cover the other parts of your path to success with clinical research.

Chapter 1:
Before you start

Find a mentor

In this chapter I will discuss ways to find a good mentor for your research period.

The first thing that you may ask may be if it is important to do research in the specific clinical area where you will be working for the rest of your life. In the very early phases of your career it may be less important to do research in the specific clinical area of your dream job than you might think. The reason for this is that your final position in the clinical area will not be judged on your specific research findings in the very early phase of your academic career but rather on later activity. So, when you are in the beginning of your academic career it is much more important that you actually *do* research – that you show activity and enthusiasm and a lot of publications. Therefore, it is not important for you to do research and to find a mentor working in your specific clinical area where you want to settle for the rest of your life. It is much more important to find a mentor that has other things to offer.

What about when you are applying for a clinical job? – Is it then important what kind of research you have done? I can tell you that this is not important. Not in the beginning of your career at least but only at a later stage. I have been head of department for some years and have employed people based on their previous academic work and the thing that you look at when you want to fill a position is mostly the activity level, not exactly what has been written in research papers but more that the applicant has actually done something - that the person has some energy and dedication for a specific area, because then you can always later change this person's focus to another clinical field. The important thing is the personality and this is judged by the activity level. Therefore, the most important thing when you apply for a job in the beginning of your career is to have a lot of papers on your publication list because that will tell the head of the department, that you have dedication and that you can actually do research.

Another issue is when you are applying for funding. Does it then matter what kind of research you have done. I will say to a certain level of course it does matter that you have done research in the specific area where you want to obtain funding, but again it is also very important that you show the funding board that you are an active person and that you have dedication and can make things happen in the academic field. That is why it is very important that you publish a lot of papers as soon as possible, because then you are in a much better position when you apply for funding for your continued research.

MENTORING

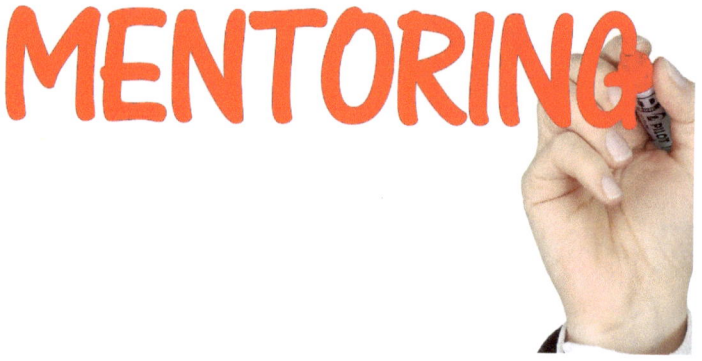

The most important thing when you choose a research area and thereby also the mentor is the mentor him- or herself. That you like this person – that you communicate well. It is much better than this person having a specific area of expertise. It is very important that you get along and can communicate with this person.

It is also important that you look at the local environment in the research group – is it a dynamic group with nice people. If this is the case then things will happen. It does not really matter so much if you have a nice table or an ugly table or a specific chair or office space. Of course you have to have office space, you have to have a place to sit and a place to work, but don't look at details. You should more look at the environment, meaning the people that you have to work with. The other researchers in the research group and of course the mentor him- or herself. So the most important factor is the chemistry.

Another very important factor is the time, meaning that your mentor has to have time for you. He or she should not be an extremely busy person that cannot talk with you more than maybe 10 minutes every month. That does not work. You have to have a person who has time for you. This does not mean that the research group has to be small. It can be a large research group because in large research groups there are very often other mentors available for daily practical problems. So, you can talk to other people in the research group about your daily problems and then at a rarer occasion you will have time together with your formal senior mentor and in these conversations you can more talk about the direction of the research and about larger problems than smaller everyday problems.

When you are looking for a good mentor then you should also realise that this mentor will actually become a kind of a friend for you. It will be your confident person, a person that you can talk with about everything, because in the research period you will also have maybe some personal problems that you need to discuss and the mentor is the person to discuss it with because if you have personal problems then the mentor has to understand that and to realise that you may not perform exceptionally well in a certain time period before you will get back on track and perform well again. So, your mentor has to be a person that you can actually talk with on every aspect of your personal life also.

Before you start you will have a conversation with the potential mentor about expectations. What do you expect from him or her? And what does the mentor expect from you? You have to be very honest here. The mentor will expect you to work maybe 40-50-60 hours a week on a specific project and sometimes evenings and nights, and if this collides with other working obligations or logistic issues in your personal life then you have to tell it and you have to agree upon your expectations, both your own and the mentor's.

In some research groups it is normal to have a formal contract where you write down all these agreements and expectations but I will say that most often this is not necessary. You have to rely on each other – you have to trust each other and if you do not do that – if you do not trust your mentor and if the mentor does not trust you, then probably this is not the place to work. So it is some kind of a dilemma here because you have to agree on your expectations and of course have to trust each other.

Occasionally, some research groups have experienced problems, especially if it is a very competitive area. The problems could for instance be who actually owns the data that you are gaining in your research project. If this becomes a problem, then I think that you should actually be quite worried and it may be time to leave. It should not be a problem at all, so if there are ownership-issues it may be a sign of potentially larger problems in the horizon. It has to be defined very clearly that you of course as a primary researcher in this field also own the data. Most often formal ownership is shared with the institution, or the institution may the formal and only owner, but ownership should never exclusively belong to the mentor. There should not be discussions here, and that has to be clear from the very beginning. You could also discuss these issues with your mentor up front before they become a problem. I think that it is quite obvious that if you for instance make a new invention in your research project then the patent will be jointly owned by you and your mentor and the institution. That is the normal way to do it and if it cannot be like that, then again I think that you should consider to change place and to find another place to work. I think that it is natural that you will be also a co-owner if you actually do the invention in your research. This applies for most academic institutions, whereas pharmaceutical companies work differently. Here the researcher will typically hand over all rights to the company where he or she is employed. In clinical research financially sponsored by a pharmaceutical company there has to be a legal and binding contract between the involved parties stating lots of different agreements including rules of ownership.

However, do not become too worried now before you have actually started. It is not a good idea to think too much about these things. Of course you have to be sure that everything works out and the chemistry between you and your mentor is probably the most important thing that you should be sure of. You have to communicate freely and in a nice fashion with your potential mentor and it has to be natural that you spend time together and actually have lots of fun.

How to get the idea for a project

Now we will discuss ways to get a good idea for a research project. It may not always be an easy task to find a great idea for your research project, so my best advice for you will be to look in your daily clinical work and then wonder. Find issues where you think "why is it so? – why are we doing things like this? Why do we give these recommendations to patients? Why do we use this kind of treatment for this kind of disease?" This is the best way to find your research question and then you will actually solve the problem when you have done your project, because the best research projects, they solve everyday problems. In your daily clinical practice you have to wonder and to ask questions all the time. It may also be a good idea to listen to the questions that are asked by for instance medical students or by the patients themselves. They may ask the right questions.

When you are doing a research project you may think that you have to first get the idea, then do the research and then write the manuscript. However, you have to look at it a little bit differently. Of course you have to start with the idea, but the next step should be to look at the manuscript outline, at least imaginary in your own brain. You have to find out how you would write an article on this issue. That will give you an idea of how to design the studies.

I can give you a good example because if for instance you are doing rounds in a surgical department and a patient has had a laparoscopic colon resection for cancer, then you have to tell this patient when he or she can go back to work, when he or she can do heavy weightlifting or run a marathon or something like that. These are natural questions for the patients and you cannot answer those questions with back-up from good scientific evidence. So you now have to find out how to answer this very relevant question from a patient. For instance, what does the restrictions that you are currently giving mean for the daily life of the patient? That could be research question number one. The research question number two could be "what is the scientific evidence behind the restrictions that you are currently giving", and question number 3 could be "what kind of information should we give to the patients in the future". What should we advise, when can they run that marathon and when can they not, and when can they go back to work. These three different research questions have now come up just by the simple question from the patient – "when can I take up my normal daily activities".

 The first research question was "what does it mean for the patient's daily life?" You can solve that or you can answer that question by a qualitative research design, for instance a focus group interview, because that will tell you what these restrictions mean for the patients in their daily life.

 The next research question was "what is the

scientific evidence for these restrictions that you are giving". That should of course be answered by a systematic review – perhaps also a meta-analysis depending on the data but at least a systematic review. For this you should follow the PRISMA-guidelines and then compose your research design as well as the final scientific paper according to these guidelines.

The third research question was "what kind of information should we give to the patients in the future?". That should ideally be solved by a randomised clinical trial where you for instance randomise patients to different kinds of advice for when to take up normal daily activities at home. You can for instance randomise to 1 week pause compared with 4 weeks pause or whatever you decide and then you can look at complications, incisional hernia development or other relevant clinical outcomes. So, ideally it should be solved by a randomised trial that should of course follow the CONSORT criteria. The CONSORT statement will guide you to the design and reporting of your randomised trial.

If this is not a possibility because it is hard work and will cost a lot of money, then you can do a more simple audit of patient files. For instance if you have one department or one hospital giving one kind of recommendation and then another hospital or another department giving another set of recommendations. Then you can compare the outcome by a retrospective study design with a simple audit of patient files. The evidence level is lower than for the randomised trial, but it may be a good compromise if do not have the time or money to perform a randomised clinical trial.

Thus, if you start with a relevant daily clinical problem, then you can design different studies. The clinical question has now become research questions suitable for more than a single study design.

This is the way to go – look in your daily clinical practice and begin to wonder and listen carefully to what questions you are asked from patients, from colleagues, and from students. Here you will find the very good research questions for your upcoming research work.

You should write a systematic review

In this chapter I will guide you through the different types of literature reviews that you can write as scientific papers. You will soon discover that I will strongly suggest that you write a systematic review within your research field and there are many good reasons for that.

First of all, a systematic review is by definition a review that attempts to collect relevant evidence that fits pre-specified criteria – this is important – pre-specified criteria to answer a specific research question. A systematic review has to have clear objectives and reproducible methodology, it has to use a systematic search for literature, it has to assess validity and bias of the included studies, and it has to use systematic presentation and synthesis of the results. All this is given in the PRISMA guidelines that you can find on the internet. The PRISMA-guidelines have been published in many different journals and the easiest way is to go to www.prismastatement.org and find all the details there.

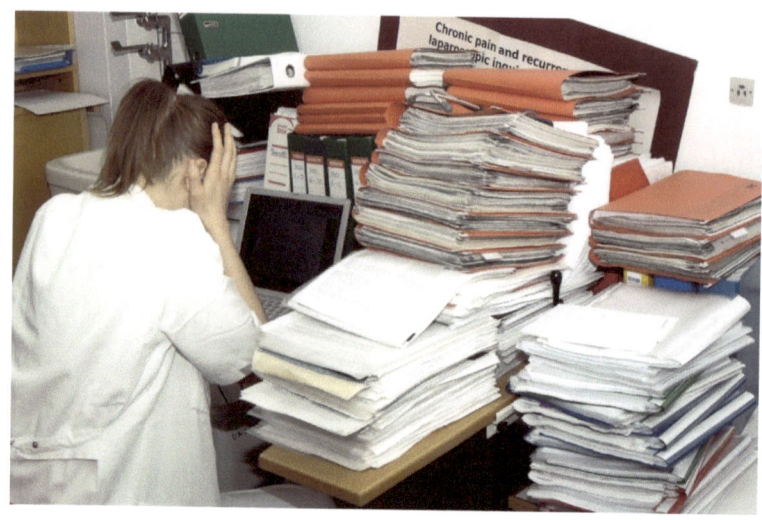

So – first of all – why write a systematic review? The main purpose is that you have a lack of knowledge within a specific field and it is an important clinical area that needs to be covered in a review. Then you have to have the time – you have to be able to invest your time to make a systematic review – and you also have to have the energy and the enthusiasm to do it. It is not a very big thing to make a systematic review, but it does take maybe a few months of work fulltime, so you have to invest the necessary time. Then it is also reasonable easy to get it published. Finally, it is important to have some successes in the start of your career, so why not do a systematic review? A positive byproduct is that when you do a systematic review within your field of research, then you also get the chance to read all the literature within your field. So it is a kind of a win-win situation, you read all the necessary literature and then also you make a good scientific paper and it is reasonably easy to get it published if it is performed well.

Narrative review

There are different types of reviews that you can write. There is the narrative review, the systematic review, the meta-analysis, and then a Cochrane review. The narrative review is as it says – a story that you tell the reader, so you do not have to make a systematic search of the literature and you can more or less choose what you want to include as references to support your message to the reader.

Systematic review

The systematic review has to use a pre-specified methodology and a pre-specified way of reporting the results. The systematic review is a kind of a qualitative synthesis of the results – this means that it presents text-based results. You are telling the reader the results in text format.

Meta-analysis

If you then do a meta-analysis which is an add-on to a systematic review then you add a quantitative synthesis on top of the systematic review and then it is called a meta-analysis. Thus, you cannot have a meta-analysis without an underlying systematic review and the meta-analysis is an add-on to a systematic review but of course within the same scientific article.

Cochrane review

Then the final form is the Cochrane review. The Cochrane review is most often a meta-analysis, but it uses a special work-flow in the writing process, so it is not just a meta-analysis. It has to follow the defined work-flow by the Cochrane collaboration. You should not be afraid of writing a Cochrane review but it should not be the first systematic review and meta-analysis that you write. In most of the Cochrane groups you will get valuable guidance in the process. One of the main differences between a "normal" meta-analysis and a Cochrane review is that you have to apply for a title of the review before you can begin. If accepted by the Cochrane Collaboration then you write a protocol that will undergo extensive peer review and if accepted it will be published. Thereafter, you can make the Cochrane review that will also undergo peer review before it can be published. If you are interested you can find detailed guidance on the Cochrane websites.

In the pyramid or the hierarchy of evidence the systematic review with homogenous randomised controlled trials and the meta-analysis are considered to be the highest level of evidence and that is evidence class 1A. The next level is 1B and this includes individual randomised trials. Evidence class 2A is also actually a systematic review, but that is a review including cohort studies and the 3A is a systematic review of case control studies. You can therefore see that the systematic review can belong to different classes of evidence with the highest possible evidence, class 1A, being a systematic review of homogenous randomised trials and a meta-analysis. Editors normally like systematic reviews because they get many citations so the impact factor of the journal will most likely increase if they print good systematic reviews in their journal.

Narrative reviews are becoming more difficult to publish. The trend in scientific biomedical publishing nowadays wants systematic rather than narrative reviews although good narrative reviews certainly have many readers. Narrative reviews are now primarily written by opinion leaders and you have to have a very good overview of the clinical field so that you are able to choose the key references yourself without a systematic literature search. So maybe the narrative review is not a good paper for you to start with. You will have to have expert knowledge within the clinical area, you have to know the clinicians' opinions about the problem in question, and you have to know the current trends and tendencies within this specific clinical field. When you do a narrative review you have to prepare thoroughly like with any scientific paper, you have to make a good and detailed outline before you write your paper. Thus, it does take some time to write a narrative review, but it does not take as much time to prepare the narrative review as it takes to prepare the systematic review or the meta-analysis. The work-load may not be so big, but again as mentioned before, it may not be the best article for you to start with because you have to be an opinion leader or at least a clinical expert within the field.

On the other hand, the systematic review does not require you to be an expert and this is actually quite interesting because normally a systematic review is considered to be a paper of very high scientific quality, but you do not have to be an expert in the specific area. You can write a systematic review almost about anything, because you follow the strict guideline within the PRISMA statement. It is quite easy to follow so you can actually write a systematic review about almost anything even though you are not an expert. So, you can easily make a systematic review also as a young researcher. When you are preparing your systematic review you have to use quite a lot of time to define your literature search, to define your data extraction. In the process you will evaluate bias and the write the qualitative synthesis according to the PRISMA guideline. The paper requires quite a bit of work from you – but as I said before – honestly, anyone can do it. So why not do a systematic review as one of your first scientific projects? The positive side for you is that you get to know the literature within your field of research and that is why I strongly advocate that a researcher that is starting within a field of research should always start with a systematic review, because it is so rewarding. You get to know the literature, it is easy to get it published if you follow the PRISMA statement thoroughly, you learn a lot about science by doing it, and it is a paper on your CV like any other papers. So that's why it is a very good idea. Furthermore, it is actually an important article to publish because you will present an overview of the field both for yourself, but especially also for the readers and then you will not waste time in your following clinical trials with designs that should not be used. That is why it is a very important paper to make early in your research career.

    It can be published both in general medical journals but also in specialised journals. If you look at the number of published systematic reviews as well as meta-analyses then the numbers are increasing exponentially through the last 10-20 years. This is of course a positive thing but it also means that it is getting harder to get your papers accepted. That is why you have to be very strict in following the PRISMA guidelines because if you do that then the likelihood of acceptance will be higher.

The meta-analysis is a quantitative add-on to the systematic review. You are not always allowed to do a meta-analysis as it depends on the data. Studies have be rather homogenous and the best way to find out if you can do the meta-analysis is to read the Cochrane hand-book. This is freely available on the internet and it is an extremely good resource, so download the Cochrane hand-book and read it from the beginning. The papers that you will put into your meta-analysis has to be similar in a way that it will be allowed to do this special kind of statistical analysis combining results across different studies.

With a meta-analysis you should pre-define the analysis plan in a kind of a research protocol, and I will suggest that you work together with a statistician who has performed meta-analyses before. This will make your life much easier. The statistician should become a co-author of your paper because the contribution of this person is substantial. It does not mean that you as the lead-author should not know anything about how to do a meta-analysis, but at least the first few times that you perform a meta-analysis you need this expert in order to actually make it happen. When you have written your meta-analysis (which includes the systematic review) and done it according to the available guidelines, it is reasonably easy to get it accepted for publication because the meta-analysis is regarded even better than the systematic review itself. Since it is normally not a problem to get it accepted for publication then why not do it if you have the time and expertise available?

In summary, it is a very good idea to make a systematic review early in your research career within your intended field of research. You will get to know the literature and it is quite easy to get it accepted for publication given that you do it the right way, and the right way is by strict following the PRISMA-guidelines. Another nice thing about the systematic review is that you do not need to be an expert within the clinical field. So why not do it? Make a systematic review.

Funding

All research projects needs funding. You may be in the situation where your mentor has already secured the necessary funding but sometimes you also have to apply yourself. This chapter will therefore try to guide you through the process of writing a good application for research funding.

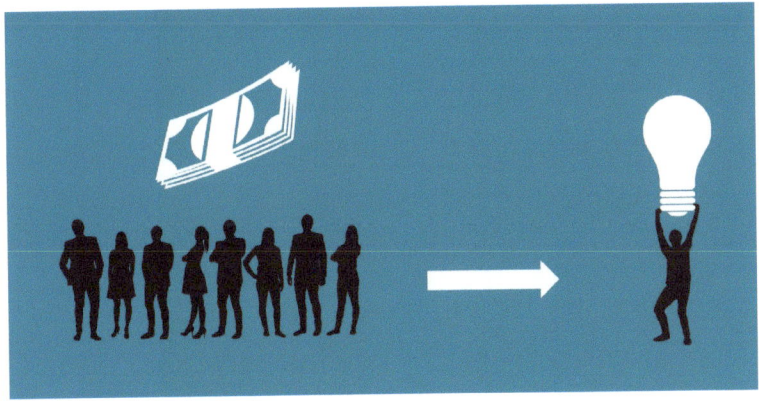

Every application has to have some kind of a cover letter. It may be very small, but it has to introduce the reader to the application. There is a human being who is actually reading your application and this person has to be introduced to your application, how much money are you requesting and for what purpose.

Then there will very often be a description of your project in layman terms, i.e. without medical terms and with no difficult words, so it has to be readable by a person not within your clinical field.

Then there of course has to be a formal description your research project. This often will cover maybe 3 to 5 pages of text including references, but that depends on where you are applying for your money, so read the application guide carefully and of course fulfil them 100%.

Then you always have to give a budget. The budget has to be detailed and with of course the correct amounts.

Then you have to supply you curriculum vitae including your list of publications. The list of publications is probably the most important part of your application. The reader will look at you as a person and decide if you are the correct person to give the money to. Will the money grow in your hands, will it be used properly and will there be some kind of output? These are the questions that you indirectly have to answer by your application and especially by your list of publications. If you have not published anything yet, then it is not likely that you get research funding and perhaps you should have your mentor make the application instead of you. But if you have some publications, then it can be a good idea for you to make the application yourself.

If you are making the application yourself there has to be some kind of a recommendation letter from both your mentor and also typically from the head of the department, because the head of the department will have to write that he or she will support you with working environment and that you actually are allowed to be there and do your research. The recommendation letter from your mentor contains other information, most importantly information about the project itself – that it is a very important project for patient care and also information about you. Her or she has to recommend you as a researcher, so that the people that are giving you the money can see that you are the right person to give the money.

Front matter
The front page of the research application can work as a cover letter. That depends on where you are applying, but you almost always have to give your contact information and inform the people

reading the application about who you are, what kind of position you have, how much money you are applying for, and if you have applied before to the same foundation and if some publications have come out of that previous donation. Then you also should write when you want to use the money, what time period, and then some foundations would like to have some key-words for indexing purposes, but that is not always the case.

In your cover letter you should explain why you are applying to this specific foundation, and why the research is important for the patients – what are the clinical implications – the perspectives of your research, because it is very important for the foundation to have this information when they discuss who they should give the money to.

Then you should also cover your practical possibilities for doing the project. For instance if you want to do a project with 10,000 patients of a certain kind and if your department only has 50 of those per year then of course you are in trouble. So, you have to explain to the foundation, that it is practically possible for you to do this research as planned and then they will see that it is a good place to put their money. You should also give information on the total financing of your study, if you are applying for a part of the financing or if it is an application for full financing. You should also give information on where they should send the money. Finally, you could also cover, but that certainly depends on the foundation, you could cover the positive effects for the foundation itself if they can use your results in a kind of commercial way to tell the World about your research and that is has been supported by this specific foundation. It is not always in the interest of the foundation to have this possibility, but is may be so.

Layman description
The next part will be the layman description and most often this should be quite short - maybe just a single page or even less. This should be a sales-pitch of your project. It should briefly explain, and without any medical terms or fancy language, why this research is important, what is the aim and most importantly, what are the perspectives for the future patient.

Project description

The next part will be the description of your project itself and if you at this stage already have made your research protocol. If you have written the protocol then it is not so difficult, because you can more or less follow your research protocol and copy-paste some of it into your application.

In this description you should divide it into different sections. First of all of course an <u>introduction</u> with your aim of study and what you want to obtain here – what information you want to obtain in your research project.

Then the <u>background</u> containing what previous evidence is available in this area, what is the clinical practice nowadays and why it could be a good idea to look at it critically and maybe change things. You could also here give the qualifications of you as a researcher and maybe also of the other participants in your research group, especially maybe the mentor could be mentioned here, that he or she is a World expert in the specific field.

The next paragraph or section could be the <u>methods</u> of your study, you should explain your study design in detail because sometimes there are people in the board of the foundation who are experts and they would like to see the detailed methods section here and then judge if you are on the right track. You should give the number of patients you want to study and especially you should also give a sample size calculation because then you can underline that you are a good researcher and have made good thoughts about this before starting the study. Of course you also have to discuss ethical issues including the different permissions that you have to obtain from the Ethics Committee and other places relevant for your study.

Typically there will also be a section about dissemination of the results. Here you will describe how you want to tell the World about your obtained results. That is of course through scientific publications, but it could also be with presentations at scientific conferences, maybe in newspaper articles, interviews and so on.

The next part of your application would be the budget and this has to be as realistic as possible and by this I mean that it is a good thing to give as exact amounts as possible. This means that you should not for instance for salary write 100,000 $

but in stead give the exact amount, e.g. 96,758 $. This will give the impression that you are sincere, that you have calculated this in detail and that you are not a liar. So give the exact amounts for the different parts of the budget and then you will gain credibility. The budget will typically have information about salary, and the running expenses should be divided into whatever is relevant. Include everything so it will become as realistic as possible.

Curriculum vitae
Your curriculum should give your contact information, your education, where you are working presently, and where you have worked previously. It could also have information on previous research funding, what conferences you have attended, what presentations you have given and then most importantly, your list of publications. Your list of publications has to be absolutely free of errors, it has to be put in the format as you will do in a scientific paper and it has to be chronological meaning that you start with number 1 with the article that was published first and then number 2 and number 3 and so on. Be

sure that you do not make any mistakes here because that will give a bad impression, so be careful with your list of publications.

You should make your curriculum pretty short and only with relevant contents and this means that if you have a full curriculum on your computer, then for every application or every time you want to use your curriculum you have to revise it to make it relevant for the specific purpose.

Letter of recommendation

The next section would be the letter of recommendation from your mentor. The mentor should here of course recommend your application, that the foundation should give you money, and this should be done by describing or explaining why the project is important. The letter of recommendation should also describe you as a person as well as a researcher, why you are the correct person to get this funding. This means that you are clever, good, hard working and maybe also lots of fun to be together with. Then finally, your mentor could also mention that the practical situation is okay, that you have the right facilities available to perform your research project.

Then there most often also should be a letter of recommendation from your head of department. This should back you up by telling the foundation that it is okay for you to be there and to perform your research at this specific institution.

Conclusion

To conclude I will say that you should read the guide from the foundation very carefully. You should start a long time before deadline, preferably maybe a month before deadline because your mentor also have to have time to read your application and to correct things before it can be submitted.

One final piece of advice: Do not ever submit a research application without approval from your scientific mentor. This is a very bad idea that you. You have to have approval every time because you are not only applying yourself, you are also actually applying on behalf of your mentor. So, you have to have approval every time.

It is good training to make a research application because it will make you think about your research and make you plan things correctly.

Prepare for the critical phases

In this chapter I will try to discuss the critical phases in the research process and how to master them.

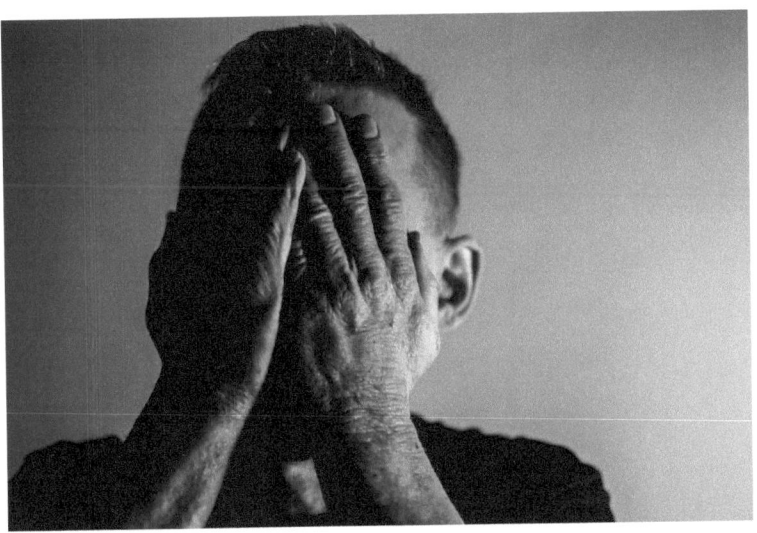

The first thing that will hit you as a young researcher is that you have to make a research protocol. So, there may be some critical phases in this research protocol writing phase and that is mainly because it will often be your first writing task and that may in itself be a little frightening. You may experience writer's block and fear of not performing well for your scientific advisor or mentor, so there are certain things here that have to be handled.

The next phase is the <u>data acquisition phase</u>. This may be prolonged - much more prolonged than you have planned it to be. It never goes the way you planned. You may have estimated how many patients you can accrue for your study within a certain time period, but this never happens. It is terrible and it is not fair but it is unfortunately often the truth. There is a law that we tend to talk about and that is Lasagna's law. Louis Lasagna was an American physician and professor of medicine and this "law" says that when you start your clinical trial, then the patients disappear. I am sorry to say, but very often that is actually true. I have no idea why it is so, but it is often the case. So you have to plan your data acquisition phase to be longer than you actually want it to be.

When you have acquired your data from your clinical trial, then the next phase will be the data <u>analysis phase</u>. This may be difficult. Very often it is driven by the p-value, i.e. you are seeking a p-value below 0.05 and of course this is the wrong way to do it. In the analysis phase you are often dependent on other researchers, on your adviser or maybe even a statistician or other people, but on the other hand it is also the climax. This is the time where you get the answer of your study – your research question. So, it is very rewarding to be in the analysis phase, but it also has some challenges.

The next phase is the <u>manuscript phase</u>, and here you have a new role if you have not written many manuscripts before. You often become the limiting factor here, because you have to produce something and you may experience pressure from your advisors or mentor or also from the co-authors.

When you have written your paper and everybody agrees to the content, it has to be submitted for publication and now you enter the <u>publication phase</u>. This is a phase where you actually cannot do anything. You have no influence on this process and very rarely it is a hole-in-one experience, meaning that it will not be accepted right away without any corrections. It often takes a long time – an extremely long time - sometimes up to a year before your paper gets published. So, you have to get used to this prolonged waiting time and it is not at all fun. The solution here is to simply do many studies, because then you always have some studies in the publication phase and some studies in other phases, but I will get back to that.

Solutions

Now I will try to touch upon some of the possible solutions. In the protocol phase you will often experience waiting time for answers from your scientific advisor, maybe from co-authors, from other collaborators, from the authorities, from the Ethics Committee etc. So, there are always waiting times in the protocol phase. That is why, if you should not become depressed and needs medication and a psychiatrist, then you have to have other tasks on your desk. You have to have other things to do and the best thing to do in the protocol phase is actually to work on for instance a systematic review.

A systematic review will take you some months to produce, and there are always some work to do in the data acquisition and analysis phases for the systematic review with article screening, bias assessment and so on, so it is a good thing to have on the side when you make your scientific protocol for your clinical trial. You can also write a case report or something else, but the important message from me to you is to have other things going on while you produce your scientific protocol.

That is why it is important as a fulltime researcher to have quite a few ongoing simultaneous research studies. These should preferably be in different phases. You have to have one study in the protocol phase, maybe one study in the data acquisition phase, one in the analysis phase, one in the writing phase, one in the publication phase and so on. This is not because you have to be pressured to produce a lot of studies. Of course that is a positive effect of it also, but the main reason for having overlapping tasks, i.e. many ongoing projects, is that you always have something to work on. You will not experience that you are just waiting and getting depressed. So, have a lot of things to do with research projects in different phases simultaneously and then you will experience a much happier workday being a researcher.

Along making a protocol you have to read the literature. This is extremely important as a researcher. You have to read both generally and also specifically within your research field. My advice to you for your general update in general biomedical science is to read some of the big general journals like The New England Journal of Medicine, The Lancet, BMJ, JAMA, and Annals of Internal Medicine. There are many to choose from, but at least those mentioned are kind of mandatory. You have to see their table of contents every week or every fortnight when they come out. You can do that quite easy by subscribing to the e-tocs (electronic table of contents). You can do that on the journals' websites by giving your e-mail address and they will send you their table of contents every time a new issue comes up. In this way you will stay updated, you can click on interesting papers and read them either as a summary or as full text, depending on your time and interest and then you will be updated.

    On top of this you also have to follow your specific research area and this can be done by screening selected journals every month when they comes out. I will advise you to make a list of journals where you need to see the table of contents every month. You can also subscribe to specific searches on PubMed. This is quite easy. Just go to the PubMed website and you can create a specific search. You have to make a user account, log-in, and then there is a place on the screen where you can subscribe to that specific search, meaning that every time a new paper comes out in your specific area, then you will get an e-mail from The National Library of Medicine.

The next phase is the <u>data acquisition phase</u>, and if you have a problem here, which I must say that almost all researchers have, then there are ways around that. The data acquisition has to be planned as detailed as possible. It is a very good idea to make a pilot patient or a few pilot patients, meaning patients where you will not use the results for anything, but you are testing your clinical set-up. You are testing how you approach the patients, how you get the data, how you monitor, how you make blood tests and so on – whatever is involved in your study. You have to have a lot of structure in the data acquisition phase. You have to be very strict on how you do things and even though you prepare it as thoroughly as you can, then very often you should increase your expected time for data acquisition. It may sometimes take twice as long as you expected. It always takes longer than you expect. It is not a catastrophe as long as you are prepared for this.

If you are performing a clinical study that is quite tough, meaning that it requires a lot of your attention and lots of practical work, it is also a good idea to put in some small time periods where you take time off of the project and do other things. The best thing to do is, as mentioned previously, to work on a systematic review.

The next phase is the <u>analysis phase</u> and this is where you have to be strict. This is where you have to stick to the plan and you will preferably have made a detailed statistical analysis plan to begin with and you simply now has to stick to the plan. It is a good idea to be in very close contact in this analysis phase with your scientific advisor and also sometimes with a statistician depending on the study design and how difficult it is.

You have to be patient in the analysis phase and it is often quite intense. You allocate all your time available for data analysis because you most often will do it within maybe a few days or few weeks and it is quite intense. This is the climax. This is where you get the answer to the research question, so it is also the time period where you have a lot of enthusiasm.

When you have analysed your results and gotten all your p-values and your major graphs and tables, then the next thing that has to happen is that you have to write the manuscript. This is called the <u>manuscript phase</u>. How to overcome the challenges in the manuscript phase is not easy, but there is very good help by doing it the same way every time. Do not invent the wheel here, you have to do it the same way every time.

I strongly suggest that you make a detailed outline of your paper in close collaboration with your author group and then when you all agree on the content, not the specific sentences but the content and direction of the paper, then you go on to the actually writing. As I will go through in detail in the next book in this series I am advocating for dictating your paper on a smartphone, but you can also write it yourself if this is what you prefer. No matter what method you use for the writing, you will have to make a detailed outline that is cleared within the author group and after that you write the paper.

This is a very good habit of scientific writing because it will solve a lot of problems. You will move a lot of work from the revision phase to the planning phase and then co-authors will not come afterwards and ask for a totally different angle on the paper because you have cleared the outline within the author group before you write the first sentence of your paper.

So, in <u>conclusion</u> you should not be worried because there are solutions for everything of course. There are some challenges in the different phases and you may call them critical phases, but they are also just simple phases of the research process and there is no reason to worry a lot about that. Be prepared for delays and be prepared for different problems and then everything will be more positive.

It is a good idea to have many ongoing projects in different phases because with this overlap you always have something to do. You will not sit around and be bored, looking out the window and be depressed. So, many projects in different phases is a good advice. When you come to the writing phase, the manuscript phase, then it is a good idea to do it the same way every time and I would advise you to make a detailed outline. Work on the outline for a long time together with your co-authors and after everybody has agreed –

then you start the writing process, and not before that.

Chapter 2: Initial study planning

Literature search for your research project

There are different ways to do this. You can of course just type in some words in PubMed or in Google and then get started, but I will try to explain why you should perform your literature search in a systematic fashion.

The reason why you should search literature systematically is that it will increase your chance of finding the relevant literature for your project, it will provide you with more robust conclusions, and it will hopefully give you more non-biased search results in your literature search.

Where to search
Now the important question is of course where you should perform your search. The most comprehensive and the largest database for literature search in the biomedical sciences is of course PubMed. On www.pubmed.com you can simply type your search terms and then you will get numerous hits. The PubMed search machine comprises more than 28 million citations for biomedical literature and these come from MEDLINE, from PubMed Central, from life

science journals and from online books. The PubMed citations and abstracts include the fields of biomedicine and health and they also cover portions of life sciences, behavioural sciences and even chemical sciences and bio-engineering. The PubMed citations come from all the journals that are indexed by MEDLINE and they come from journals and manuscripts that are deposited by the publishers in PubMed Central, and you also get hits from the NCBI bookshelf - that means full text books.

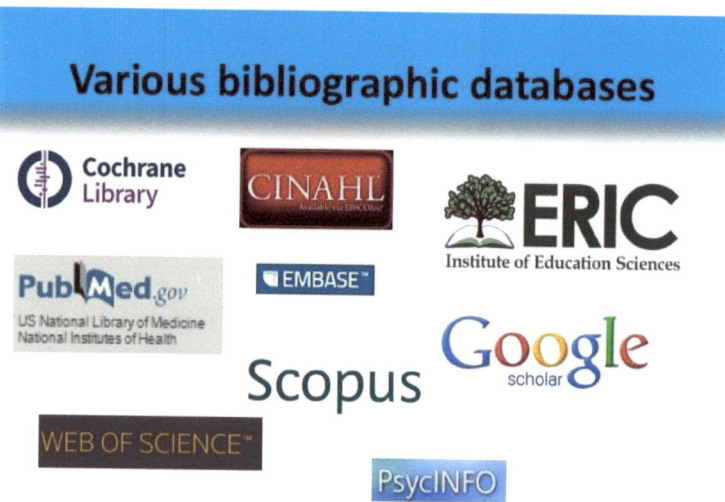

Even though PubMed is the largest database for you, there are numerous other places that you can perform your literature search. You can search in the Cochrane Library, you can search in Cinahl, Embase, Eric, Scopus, Google Scholar, Psycinfo, Web of Science and many more. Some of these have substantial overlap, but you will also find literature in one database that you will not find in other databases. There are many databases out there that can provide you with references for your research paper and also for your background knowledge for your project.

The Cochrane library has indexed many randomised clinical trials and of course their own Cochrane reviews. Most of the material in the Cochrane Library is also available in PubMed, because all the randomised trials are published in indexed journals, and most if not all of the Cochrane reviews will also be available in PubMed.

Most researchers also use Embase. Embase is a database of literature and is run by the publisher Elsevier and Embase has currently about 32 million records. They include over 8,500 journals from over 95 countries, including MEDLINE titles, and over 2,900 indexed journals unique to Embase. One of the main advantages with Embase is the export option, which is quite good. You can easily export citations to for instance an Excel sheet or other formats and you can yourself choose which fields you want to export. So you can for instance in Embase choose to export the abstract, the authors, language, or whatever you want to get out into your Excel sheet.

Export options in PubMed

Export options in PubMed are not as good as in Embase. Here you can only choose to send it to a textfile, a txt-file, you can send it to something they call collections, order, citation manager, clipboard, to an e-mail or to your own bibliography. However, it is not so easy to export it directly to an Excel sheet, but there is another solution for this (PubMed2XL - see below).

Web of Science

In Web of Science you can also search literature, but I am not sure that it will actually provide you with many more useful hits. If you are performing a systematic review in the biomedical sciences, then you are to a large extend covered by the other databases. However, it seems that Web of Science covers also papers that are much older than the papers in PubMed, so if you are looking specifically for older literature then Web of Science may be the place for you to go.

The number of journals that are covered by PubMed is around 6,000 and in Web of Science it is about 8,700 and in Scopus, which is another place to search literature, they are actually covering about 13,000 journals. The period covered in PubMed is 1950 to present, in Scopus it is 1966 to present and in Web of Science it is 1900 to present.

"Similar articles"

When you are searching for literature, not in the systematic fashion but when you are surfing on the web, it is very usable to use the function "similar articles" in PubMed. That is when you find a paper in PubMed, then on the right side of the screen there is a list of "similar articles".

Grey literature

Then you should also consider, depending on your ambitions for the systematic review, to search for "grey" literature. Grey literature is literature that is not formally published in sources such as books or journal articles. It has been said that some years ago about 10% of the references in Cochrane reviews were actually from grey literature. So, it can be a good idea to look for "grey" material if you want to make a very comprehensive systematic review. For this purpose there is a place called "Open Grey" (www.opengrey.eu) as well as numerous other local databases. If you want to include grey literature in your systematic review it is highly recommendable to get help from a professional research librarian (information specialist).

Snowball search

The next important tool for searching literature is something called "hand search". That means that you go through the reference lists of the paper that you have found already and then find relevant new material. It is also called "snowballing". This means that you find a reference maybe in one paper, you go to that, and then you find another reference in that reference list, and that is the snowball that is running down the hill. It is a very important supplement to the electronic searches and amazingly enough, even though the electronic databases are fantastic, then you will find further material by snowballing. You have to monitor how many papers you are getting by the snowballing, because that number has to go into your PRISMA-flowchart when making your figure 1 in your systematic review.

Unpublished trials
If you want to be really comprehensive and make the best systematic review, then you should also search for ongoing and unpublished but finished trials. This can be done by going to the public registries, where trials are mandatory to be registered around the World.

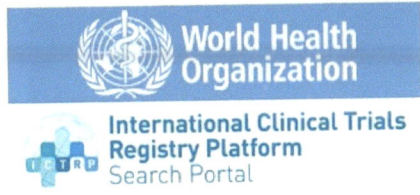

http://apps.who.int/trialsearch/

There are many of these registries – and the 17 largest deliver data to the International Clinical Trials Registry Platform (ICTRP). This is one single searchable database. You go to the World Health Organisation Clinical Trials Registry Platform and the web-address is apps.who.int/trialsearch. Here you will find data from all the approved registries. Many of them provide data once a week and some of them data every 4 weeks to this WHO trial search platform.

When to search
Now, when should you actually search literature in the research process? You have to do this several times along the way. When you are getting the idea for your project, then you will have to look into the literature to find out if it is a feasible project. Is it interesting, and what has been done previously within this research area. So, you will do a non-systematic search at this point. You will then get a good idea if evidence is lacking and you will develop your hypothesis by doing this initial non-systematic surfing in the literature databases.

When you have developed your PICO and are ready for the correct and final systematic literature search, then it is a good idea, at least when you are doing a systematic review and meta-analysis, to get professional help from an information specialist. They are very skilled and can search in several databases and deep the final search string in a way that will give you more relevant and less irrelevant hits.

Boolean operators

In all systemic searches the so-called "Boolean Operators" will make it possible to combine different search terms in the same search string. The three basic boolean operators are AND, OR and NOT. For instance in PubMed, if you are searching for circulating cells, you will get 79,378 hits. If you search for the word "tumor" then you will get more than 3.5 million hits. So if you combine these 2 searches for "circulating cells" and "tumor" with the boolean operator AND, then your result will only be about 26,000 hits because the terms circulating cells and tumor have to be present at the same time in every single hit. Instead, if you use the boolean operator OR between circulating cells and tumor, then it will boost your results to more than 3.5 million hits because any paper that has either circulating cells or tumor in it will come up in your search results. The term NOT is used less often. If you write "circulating cells NOT tumor" then it will give you all the papers with circulating cells, but it will subtract the papers that has the word tumor in it. So the result will be only about 52,000 hits.

Asterix

You will also often use an asterix (*) in your search string. This can be a powerful tool because it will expand your search to include all the different endings on a certain word. For instance, if you put chemotherapy* instead of chemotherapy then you in PubMed will get 175 different search terms with OR as a boolean operator between them. This is done automatically by PubMed.

Use of asterix (*) in PubMed

chemotherap*

- chemoterapeutic[All Fields] OR
chemoterapeutical[All Fields] OR
chemoterapeuticka[All Fields] OR
chemoterapeuticke[All Fields] OR
chemoterapeuticky[All Fields] OR
chemoterapeutics[All Fields] OR
chemoterapeutiese[All Fields] OR
chemoterapeutik[All Fields] OR ......

Quick and dirty

There is also something called a "quick and dirty" search. This is when you simply type a few words in the search field in PubMed and then PubMed will provide you with lots of different options, lots of different searches actually, within this quick and dirty search. For instance if you put the words "robot surgery", then it will give you all kinds of different combinations. It will search on robot, it will search on surgery, it will search on surgical procedures, operative, and many more. This will cover many different combinations and it will give you many hits even though you have put only the words "robot surgery" in the search field.

However, this is not a systematic literature search, so it is only used in the beginning when you are surfing the area on PubMed with a quick and dirty search.

Block search

When building a search string it is usual to use so-called "block search". A block search is when you divide your research question into different parts and then you search every block or every part by itself, and then in the end you combine the different searches. For instance – if you have a research question, that is "are circulating tumor cells increased in the blood in patients with primary liver cancer", then you could divide this search into 3 different blocks: liver cancer, circulating cells, and blood. So now you will take every block by itself, for instance in the liver cancer block you can search for "liver neoplasm", combine it with the boolean operator OR to "hepatocellular cancer" or "liver cancer" or "hepatic cancer" just to give an example. Then this combined search with OR in between for liver cancer – that comprises one search in the end and that can later on be combined with the other blocks. The circulating cells block could consist of a search for "tumor embolic cell", "blood cell", "tumor cell circulating", and "tumor embolism" and these individual searches should be combined with OR in between. The blood block could be "hematologic test" or "blood test" or "blood specimen collection" or blood sample and then they will be combined together to one single search result. Then in the end you will combine these 3 blocks with the boolean operator AND in between and you will have a combined search result that will provide you with hopefully the answer to your research question whether circulating tumor cells are elevated in the blood in patients with primary liver cancer. As you can see it is actually not so simple to build your search string using this different blocks and again I would strongly advice for you to get help from a research librarian because they know the skills here – they know how to build your search string in the correct manor so it will cover all the required questions.

PubMed2XL
The next problem is that you have to export your search from PubMed to for instance an Excel file

or to another way of looking at your search result. If you are using PubMed, then it is actually not so easy to export the result to Excel, but there is a solution for this problem. A brilliant guy has developed a small shareware (free) program, and you can find it on the web-address: http://blog.humaneguitarist.org/projects/pubmed2xl/ Here you can download the exe file and that will solve your problem. Using this program you can export your search results into an Excel sheet and you can now sort the references, you can exclude doublets and you can do lots of things.

blog.humaneguitarist.org/projects/pubmed2xl/

Covidence

If you are making a systematic review you can also use the newer program at Covidence. The address is covidence.org. This is developed by the Cochrane collaboration and the trick here is to export your search into a reference manager and then from the reference manager software you can export it into Covidence. Covidence is a very nice tool. It is easy to use when you are screening the articles and select which will be included and excluded for the upcoming data extraction process.

Covidence.org

Covidence is currently free for one review with 2 reviewers and after that there is a fee. It is very important in the screening process to be careful about what you are actually doing, because you have to put all the numbers in your figure 1 in your systematic review - the so-called PRISMA flowchart. So we have to know exactly how many hits you got from PubMed, from Embase, from Cochrane and how many hits you got from your snowball search. Thereafter, the number of excluded doublets, and the number of excluded papers for various reasons. So you have to be careful and know exactly how many papers that go in and out of your systematic review along. In the final article this process is shown in the PRISMA flowchart as figure 1. The tools for this are either Excel or Covidence – everything else is a lot of work.

Conclusion

It is advisable to get help from a professional librarian and do not only use single words in your search. You will build a complicated search string using block searches with multiple boolean operators, and the final complicated search string will be published in your systematic review.

Choose the best study design

The classical pyramid of evidence defines that the highest level of evidence can be obtained by a systematic review with or without a meta-analysis. Then the randomised controlled trials is the next level followed by cohort studies, case controlled studies, case series and case reports and the lowest evidence level is for editorials and expert opinions.

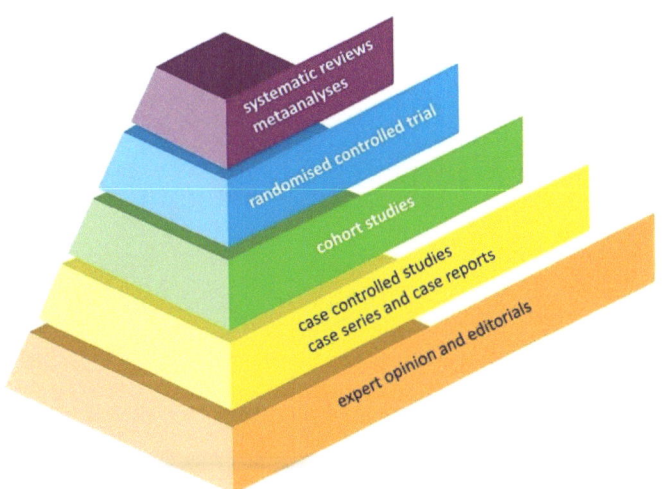

Before considering a clinical study it is advisable to do a <u>systematic review</u>. This is a very good exercise and it is fairly simple because you have good support in the PRISMA-guidelines. You will also when making the systematic review automatically be updated in your field of research so it is positive on more than one level.

If you have done your systematic review and decided on gathering clinical data, then you have to decide on the study design. There are many factors involved in the decision of what kind of study you can do and of course the best would do a <u>randomised controlled trial</u>, but very often this is not possible. There could be issues of funding (because a randomised controlled trial cannot be performed without often quite extensive external funding). Sometimes, the research question may not be optimally answered by a randomised controlled trial, so other study designs may also be considered.

In a <u>cohort study</u> you will prospectively expose a group of patients to a certain treatment. Then you are following these patients and will thereby be able to evaluate the effect of the intervention but without a control-group. It is possible to have a historical control-group for cohort studies, but it does not make it a randomised clinical trial.

There is actually a study design in between and that is the <u>quasi-randomised trial</u>. This means for instance that you can include the intervention group in one institution and the control group (prospectively) in another institution. You could also include all intervention patients on one weekday and all the control patients on another weekday. If you in this way do not randomise patients by the usual "lottery" method, but still have a control group that you cannot on purpose include with a bias, then it can be called a quasi-randomised trial. This can be a good option depending on your local issues of feasibility.

An important quality parameter in a randomised clinical trial is that you do an actual randomisation and this will in the optimal setting result in no differences in baseline characteristics. If you want to perform a quasi-randomised trial, then the same issues is important meaning that you can only do the quasi-randomised design if it is reasonable to expect that the baseline characteristics in the two patient groups will be the same. This means that if you include the intervention group in one institution and the control group in another institution, then you cannot do this in a quasi-randomised design if the patient characteristics are highly different between the two populations. For instance you cannot have your control group from rural Africa and your intervention group from a Manhattan Hospital.

Another option is to do a <u>case-control study</u> and in this study design you are comparing patients with a certain disease (the cases) with a healthy control group (the controls). Typically, you will look back in time in a so-called respective design to identify risk factors. This is also called a retrospective cohort and the retrospective cohort could constitute your control group and the prospective cohort could constitute your cases.

When we now climb down the ladder of evidence then the next study design will be the <u>case series</u> (more than 2 cases) or the <u>case report</u> (1-2 cases). In this study design you simply describe a very small cohort of patients in either the case series or the case-report. You will only be able to publish a case series or case report if there are specific learning points for the reader. These papers are still important and most brilliant ideas for new treatments and discovering of diseases are based on such publications originally.

The above mentioned study designs are mostly aimed at the quantitative research traditions. There are numerous study designs in the qualitative research traditions including questionnaire studies, focus group interviews, field studies etc. This is however out of scope of the present book to describe these study designs in detail.

Feasibility

When you have your brilliant research idea and are full of energy, then before you start writing a study protocol or make other detailed preparations, it is important to consider the feasibility of the study. This means you have to consider the different possible obstacles for the practical parts of the study.

First of all, it is a good idea to consider the <u>length of time necessary</u> to do the study. If you work for instance in an institution where they only operate 20 gastric bypasses per year and you want to randomise 2 x 500 patients, then of course the feasibility does not look very good.

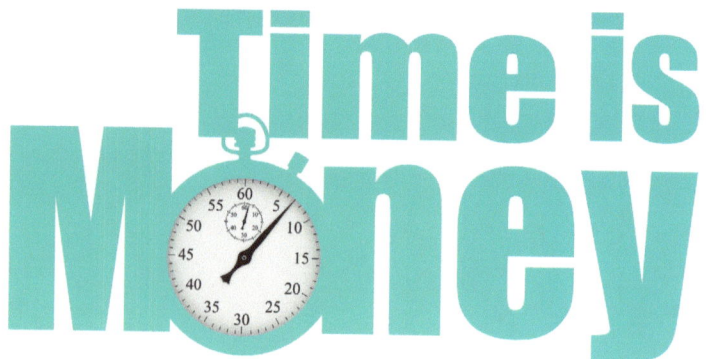

It is often the case that when you start patient accrual then somehow the patients will disappear. This is a strange phenomenon and is called "Lasagna's law". It was one of the pioneers in clinical pharmacology, the American Louis Lasagna, who described in 1970 a common phenomenon in clinical trials: The incidence of patient availability sharply decreases when a clinical trial begins and returns to its original level as soon as the trial is completed. Therefore, it is important to be conservative when planning a clinical trial. In practical terms that means, that when you have considered the necessary time for patient accrual you should probably double that estimate.

Other factors to consider are the <u>ethical</u> constraints, and if you are not a very experienced clinical researcher it would be a good idea to discuss the ethical issues with your scientific mentor early in the planning phase. It might be straight forward, but if there are potential problems, then it is important to take those into account as early as possible in the planning phase.

Nowadays, it is almost impossible to perform a research study on your own. You need the

<u>cooperation</u> with others and this has to be considered carefully because you will be the only one who have a burning desire to complete the study so the cooperation with others will most often need your attention in all phases of the trial. You need to be very active to follow-up on your co-workers and to motivate them to perform optimally.

    The next thing is the <u>cost</u> issue. This is of course very important and you need to find the necessary funding before you can start the study. For smaller simple trials it may sometimes be performed without external funding, but a larger interventional

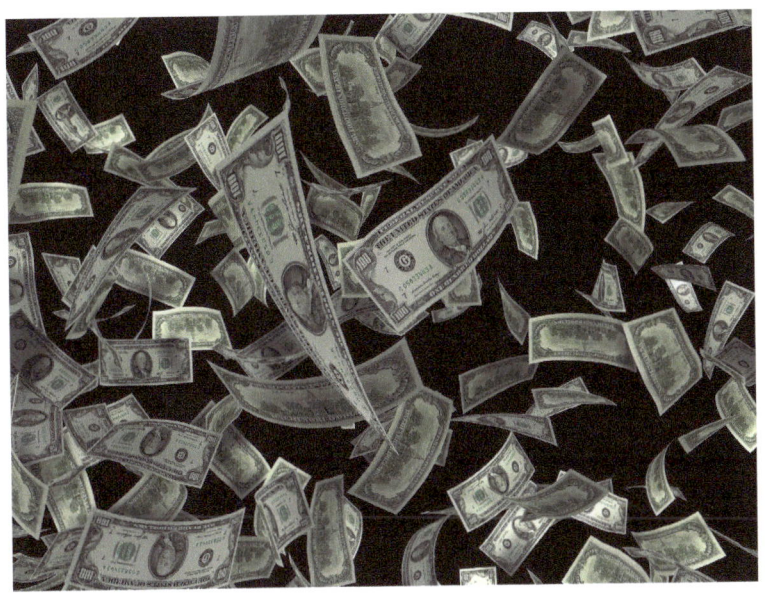

trial will most often need extensive funding before it can be realistically done in a busy clinical department.

Finally you can consider your <u>own skills</u>, meaning that you should think it through carefully if you can handle all the necessary parts of the trial with your own skills. You will as mentioned above of course have co-workers but try to write down a list of necessary skills for your study and then you can see if all the skills are covered by either you or the co-workers. If there are uncovered skills, then you simply have to include the necessary people in your list of co-workers.

Finally, I will advise you to have a close dialogue with your <u>head of department</u> early on in the planning phase. There may be structural changes underway that you don't know about and it is imperative to have the support, both morally and financially from your chief, so go and present your idea and inform him or her about the plans.

Good Clinical Practice

In chapter I will discuss the Good Clinical Practice guidelines that are implemented in many parts of the World and are mandatory in The European Union. These rules are very important to know about because you cannot perform any interventional trials with pharmacological agents or devices without following these rules of Good Clinical Practice.

> **Good Clinical Practice = GCP**

In Europe it started with a directive from The European Union some years ago and then this directive was lifted to become national laws in all the member countries of the Union. So now it is mandatory by law to follow these guidelines. In the US and other parts of the World the same rules are in effect but there may be some minor differences in the details, and the legal basis is named differently. The essence is however the same in almost all parts of World because regulatory authorities follow more or less the same criteria when applications for new drugs are considered. The overall purpose is of course to increase the quality of the studies and also of course increase data integrity.

These rules originally came out of something called The International Council for Harmonisation of Technical Requirements for Pharmaceuticals for Human Use, the so called ICH (www.ich.org). The members of this group are the European Union, Japan, United States, Canada, Switzerland, Brazil, China, Singapore and Korea.

From the researcher's point of view the main thing in these guidelines is that you have to have very good control of all the documents in your study, you have to create a trial master file (TMF), you have to use case report forms (CRFs) and the study has be monitored by an external monitor.

Trial Master File = TMF

In the trial master you will keep all essential documents for the study. This means that you keep all versions of the study protocol, all versions of the CRF and you keep an updated list of all the persons involved in the project including their curriculum vitae as well as documentation that they are familiar with the Good Clinical Practice guidelines. Then you have to have all the correspondence and the permissions from the ethical committee (IRB), various regulatory agencies and institutions, registrations, and copies of all agreements, contracts between sponsors and investigators or sponsor or the pharmacy or a pharmaceutical company, meaning every available contract that has something to do with the study should be included in the trial master file. Then you have to include your study budget, your written information sheet for the patients, the informed consent form, and all the various questionnaires and other documents that the patients are given during the study. Then everything you have about the study medicine meaning all the documents from the pharmaceutical company, from the pharmacy, and from everybody involved in the process. Then you have to give information about all the analyses and investigations that the patients are going through in the study and also detailed information of how you will handle adverse events, meaning when to contact the sponsor and when to contact the authorities. Finally, you will also of course include all the correspondence and the contract with the local GCP Unit that will most often take care of the monitoring of the study. If you don't have a local GCP Unit to do that, then it is probably an external clinical research organisation (CRO), which is a privately owned company, that will take care of the monitoring of the study.

 Thus, the trial master file may be quite extensive and usually it is required that you have all these documents on paper. In many countries it is allowed to have an electronic trial master file in stead. If required on paper, then the actual trial master file in a separate binder has be secured in a locked cabinet so it will not disappear. You will of course also have an electronic copy of the trial master file and whether the CRO or the local GCP Unit requires the electronic version or the paper version may depend on local traditions and regulations.

> **Case Report Form = CRF**

The next thing according to Good Clinical Practice is that you have to have a Case Report Form for every case, meaning every patient that will enter your trial. This is actually a really good advice, not only for GCP regulated trials, but for all trials that you are performing in your research career. Always make a formal CRF because it will help you immensely during the phase with data gathering as well as in the analysis phase. If you are doing a GCP regulated trial, then the CRF has to fulfil certain rules and you will have to study that in detail on websites of the GCP unit that you will be using. In summary the CRF has to have clearly defined areas where you can put your data with no possibility of misinterpretation and if you have put a wrong number for instance in a field in the CRF, then you are not allowed just to wipe it out and write something else. You have to cross it and then write the date of correction and your initials and then write the correct value. So, there are certain rules how to handle the CRF and they are all part of the GCP regulations.

When you make a CRF, then it is a good idea to make it as extensive as possible meaning that you have to include everything that you can think of in the study. This includes e.g. the exclusion and inclusion criteria so you can simply tick them off when you are screening a patient for inclusion in the trial. Then of course all the variables that you have to obtain for your study and then also some pages that will cover premature exclusion of a patient during the study.

Most often, the CRF is on paper, but it can also be electronic, especially in the larger pharma-driven trials. The electronic solution is expensive but has certain advantages especially in multicenter trials. It is also helpful for the researcher because you don't have to have all these papers lying around in your office. Whether electronic or on paper the content is exactly the same of course. If it is on paper you will have a binder (CRF) for every single patient that enters the study and this binder will follow the patient throughout the study period and in the end you will hand over this binder to the CRO who will take care of the further analysis, or if it is your own trial then you will use this CRF to transfer the data to for instance an Excel sheet or a statistical analysis program for data analysis.

After the trial you have to save the CRFs for maybe up to 15 years but it depends on local regulations, so you have to check that in detail before you put them away for storage.

Good Clinical Practice is mandatory by law in most countries and it involves a trial master file (TMF), a monitoring plan for external monitoring, and case report forms (CRFs) for every patient. The practical work during data acquisition in the trial is heavily regulated by these rules and therefor you of course have to know about it and to follow them to the point.

Chapter 3:
Now it is getting serious

The research protocol

There are different types of research protocols. Typically, we think of two different types and that is the very large one for the clinical trials and smaller protocols for other types of studies.

The large standard protocol
The large version has to follow certain rules. First of all you will give your study an informative title. It has to be the full title and very often it will also have an acronym which makes it much easier in daily clinical practice when talking about your study with co-workers, nurses or patients.

Then very often the research protocol will have a synopsis in the beginning because the protocol itself may be a quite lengthy document, so it is a good idea to have a small synopsis in the beginning of the protocol.

The next paragraph should be the background. In the background section you will go through the literature in detail with references along the way and you will discuss what has been shown already and where research is lacking, so in that way you will argue for your current study.

The next section is the aim of study that has to have its own separate paragraph with a headline saying "Aim of study" and here you will give your aim, preferably as short as possible in order for the reader of the protocol to understand it very easily.

The next section is of course the largest one and that is the methods section. In the methods section you will go through your study step by step. The easiest thing is to do it in chronological order meaning what has to happen first, then second and so on, with the patients. You will also give inclusion and exclusion criteria in this section. Be as detailed as you possibly can here because the methods part of the protocol is the most important part. You will also use this later when writing your paper (especially the methods section).

The next paragraph could be data-management, covering how data will be managed, the way it will be stored securely, and the rules for data access and data sharing. Many journals now demands a data sharing statement when submitting a scientific original article, so you might as well think it though already in the protocol. This is advisable because you may have to ask for a specific permission from the individual patient at inclusion, and thereby have it mentioned specifically in the written patient information and approved by the ethics committee.

The next section could be about <u>side-effects</u>. This section should describe in detail how you will handle possible side effects. There are certain rules for this and the GCP monitor can often help you to write this section in the protocol. There are standard phrases that can be used and then adapted to your specific study.

The next section typically is about <u>sample size</u>. You will have to calculate your needed sample size in order for your hypothesis to be tested. In this context I will strongly advocate for making also a formal statistical analysis plan. I know that this is not usual in a research protocol, and it is much more usual in a protocol article if you are making such a paper, but a statistical analysis plan is a very good exercise for you to do because then you will later on have to stick to your analysis plan and you cannot go on fishing expeditions in your data set. So make a statistical analysis plan in your protocol.

The next paragraph could be about <u>monitoring</u> of the study and that is especially relevant if you have a study that has to follow GCP-guidelines because then you have to write something about monitoring of the study.

The next section could be ethics and other permissions, and registration in internet databases. You will write where the study will be registered and if possible also give the exact registration numbers.

The next section typically would be budget and financing, who is sponsoring your study with money and what the money should be used for.

The next section could be some thoughts about how to tell the world about your results. You will here state if the results will be submitted to a peer reviewed scientific journal, which news media you will approach after publication (if any) and so on. Many funding agencies require details about dissemination of results, so you might as well think it through and at least suggest something here.

Finally, you will give literature references especially to your background section in the protocol.

After these sections, you will typically have a section about the criteria for information of the patient, including on the environment that the information be given in, will there be time for the patient to think about it (typically 24 hours if it is a non-urgent clinical trial), and can they have another person present for this information meeting.

Then there will be a written <u>informed consent form</u> that has to comply with specific rules, and these rules are different from country to country because of the different ethical committee systems around the World. This written informed consent form can often also be based on a standard template that you most probably can obtain from the GCP-monitor.

Other types of protocols

There are other types of protocols that you can make and these are typically made for systematic reviews, for observational studies, for quality assurance studies, for retrospective studies, for register studies and so on. These smaller protocols will much more focus on the methods section and thereby they will more function as a work plan or a detailed to do list during the actual study phases.

Who is it for?

The research protocol has to be submitted to the Ethics Committee or the Institutional Review Board or whatever it is called in your country. The protocol will also be evaluated by the National Medicines Agency (or similar), the GCP-unit, the funding agency, and all the different collaborators that you get in touch with during the process - especially before study start. Also the sponsors of the study – the ones that will actually pay the money – they of course will need a detailed research protocol in order to decide if they can support you or not.

On the PROSPERO database for registering systematic reviews they do not need a detailed protocol but they will need some information that you will take from your research protocol. This is similar to the trial registration websites such as clinicaltrials.gov where they do not need the actual protocol, but they will need some information from the protocol itself.

Thus, there are may good reasons to make a detailed research protocol and most importantly you write the protocol for yourself. During the study you may consult the protocol several times if you forget details in the study design. We are all just human beings and some clinical trials will run for years and along the way I can assure you that you will forget some details about the study. So make a detailed research protocol for your own sake and also for the different stakeholders involved and also do yourself a favour and make a detailed statistical analysis plan already before you include the first patient.

The statistical analysis plan

The purpose of making a statistical analysis plan is to lock the planned data analyses prior to analysing the first outcome parameter.

This means, that you have in advance thought everything through in detail and planned all your analyses including how you want to present your data in figures and tables. Optimally, this should be done prior to inclusion of the first patient.

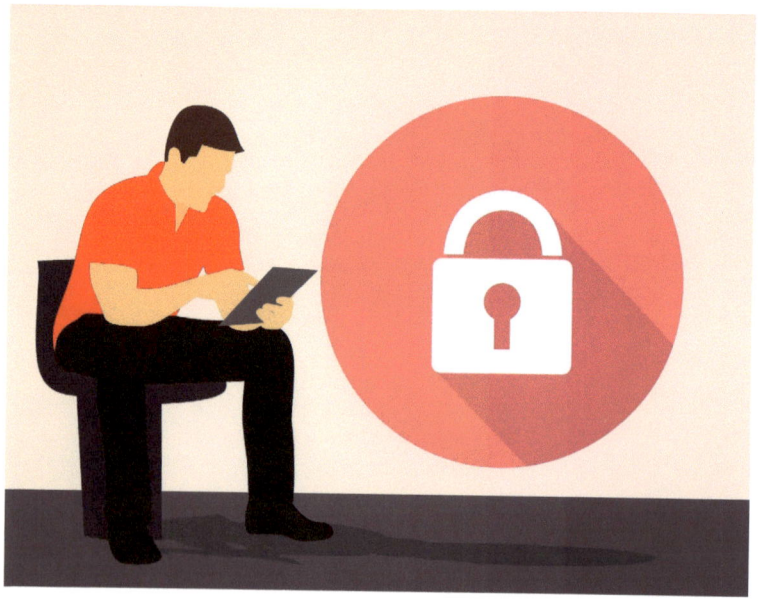

When you have decided on your statistical

analysis plan then the document should be dated and locked. In this way you are not able to go on fishing expeditions in your data analyses afterwards and this is scientifically the optimal method. If you however, later in your data analyses suddenly get a good idea for additional (exploratory) analyses then you are of course allowed to do so, but it cannot be part of your conclusion in the paper. The conclusion should strictly adhere to the aim of study and thereby the pre-planned statistical analyses.

It is not yet mandatory that you submit a statistical analysis plan together with the submitted manuscript, but some of the big journals will regard the submission of a statistical analysis plan as a positive parameter in the overall evaluation of your scientific paper. It is therefore advisable to produce a detailed statistical analysis plan whenever it is possible for you. I would say that it is <u>always</u> possible and you might as well get the habit of working with statistical analysis plans for all your studies.

A typically statistical analysis plan will cover around 5-10 pages of text and if you make it in a Word document you can convert it to a pdf-file and lock it for instance as an "image pdf-file". In this way it is not possible to alter the text afterwards and dated and a locked image pdf-file is a good proof for the editor of the journal that you have followed one of the best possible ways of conducting research.

Composition of the statistical analysis plan
The first part is a short <u>introduction</u> where the clinical problem is briefly described. It should in no way be as lengthy as the introduction section in the research protocol since the statistical analysis plan should be regarded as a supplement to the protocol. In this section you may typically start by saying that the current document is the final statistical analysis plan covering the study named xxx with the trial registration number xxx.

 The next paragraph could be the analysis <u>objective</u> followed by <u>hypothesis</u>, definition of <u>analysis sets/population/subgroups</u>. Then you typically will define your variables in end-points clearly stating your <u>primary and secondary outcome parameters</u>.

 The next paragraph could be called "<u>derivation of end-points</u>" and will explain the nature of your end-points, e.g. the nature of the data and how they are measured.

Depending on the study design, then you could have sections explaining <u>explanatory variables</u> and <u>confounder variables</u>, so that you will mention and define all the variables that will later on be included in the detailed analyses.

It is mandatory to include a section of how you will handle <u>missing values</u> and this section should in detail describe your method of data imputation or whatever system you will employ for handling of missing values.

Then the <u>statistical methodology</u> will be explained in detail including the <u>type of analyses</u>, the <u>presentation of results</u> and the original <u>sample-size calculation</u>.

Then you in detail will describe how you will <u>analyse your primary and secondary end-points</u>. This description is much more detailed than the short description that you may have mentioned in your study protocol or registered on a trial registration website. This means that you to the smallest detail will describe which variable will be tested with which method against which other variables and what kind of statistics you will use.

This section is the most important section of your statistical analysis plan and should be quite elaborate. In this way you will settle your planned statistical analyses before you make any calculations. This is the important aim of the statistical analysis plan.

The next section could define what figures you will have in your final scientific paper and what tables you want to produce. The description of figures and especially tables should include definition of exactly what variables to include and how detailed you want to describe them in figures and tables.

The final section of the statistical analysis plan could be a list of references depending on what you have described in the document. Often it is necessary to give the references to papers covering the planned statistical analyses.

What happens with the analysis plan?
In the final manuscript in the methods section you will describe that the a statistical analysis plan was made before analysing any of the data and you can supply the statistical analysis plan as a supplementary file for web publication only or at

least for the editor and peer reviewers to see when evaluating your manuscript. This means that you will typically upload the statistical analyses plan in the electronic manuscript submission system as an additional file.

In the cover letter to the editor it is advisable to describe this and suggest that the statistical analysis plan could be published as supplementary web-only file or at least the editors and peer reviewers can see it when evaluating your manuscript.

The authorship contract

When you participate in large multicenter clinical trials then the issue of authorship is of course important. Very often there may be hundreds of contributors to a clinical trial especially in the data acquisition phase, and of course all those people cannot be offered authorship. So you need to settle this issue as early as possible.

Contract of authorship
I have had some experience with an authorship contract which can actually solve many of these disputes and problems before they arise. It is a good idea to define before the study starts who will be offered formal authorship according to the ICMJE authorship criteria. This means that the persons that you define as potential authors, they will be invited to participate in the writing and revision phase of the manuscript and of course also provide final approval before submission. You have to be realistic because you cannot offer authorship to hundreds of people because they will simply not fulfil the authorship criteria at the end.

You see sometimes in the literature that

people use group names as author names. I think that that is actually a bad idea because you are either an author or you are a contributor. You cannot participate in a group author name and not fulfil the authorship criteria. It is either or. So there is no quick fix here – you simply have to fulfil the authorship criteria in order to be an author so why not simply put all the names in the byline.

That brings us back to the issue of who will be offered authorship when the study is finished. Normally it is not a problem to fulfil the first authorship criterion because that concerns data acquisition. But then, who will move on to be invited into the writing or revision phase. If the study involves numerous clinical departments for instance, then it can be a solution if you define up front that each department may send one or two persons to participate as formal authors during the writing process. It can also be defined as a minimum number of accrued patients for a study or you can use maybe other criteria as long as you define it before the study starts.

Typically, in these large trials, there will be a pre-defined (pre-defined in the protocol) writing group consisting of for instance the lead author and also a senior author that typically is placed at the end of the byline and then maybe 3, 4 or 5 additional persons. On top of that you have to decide who will additionally be invited from each participating center and this should be written in an authorship contract that should be signed by all participating centers before the study starts.

We have published a paper on this issue in 2015 in The Danish Medical Journal and the citation is "Dan Med J 2015;62(2):A5009". You can find it on PubMed and on the Danish Medical Journal's website. An example of an authorship contract is given in this publication and reproduced here, as it is an open access publication:

APPENDIX A

Authorship contract

Project name:

_____

Date:

The ICMJE recommends that authorship is based on the following four criteria:

- Substantial contributions to the conception or design of the work; or the acquisition, analysis or interpretation of data for the work; AND
- Drafting the work or revising it critically for important intellectual content; AND
- Final approval of the version to be published; AND
- Agreement to be accountable for all aspects of the work in ensuring that questions related to the accuracy or integrity of any part of the work are appropriately investigated and resolved.

All those designated as authors shall meet all four criteria for authorship, and all who meet the four criteria shall be identified as authors. Those do not meet all four criteria shall be acknowledged as contributors, typically in the acknowledgements section in the manuscript.

If a group-name is used in the byline, then typically a footnote and the acknowledgement section shall clearly state who are regarded (and indexed) as authors and who shall be regarded (and indexed) as contributors. Other terminology such as protocol committee, writing committee etc. may be misleading for the indexing process and it is highly recommended only to use the terms authors and contributors stating exact names for the persons involved.

In large multi-centre trials, numerous persons will typically be involved in ICMJE-authorship criterion one, e.g. acquisition of data. The present authorship contract designates the criteria for these persons to be offered participation in authorship criteria two, three and four, thus who will be included in the manuscript preparation to an extent that they will qualify to be an author instead of a contributor.

It is the responsibility of the first author, if applicable, to involve all co-authors to an extent that they fulfill all four authorship criteria.

First author:

Last author:

Predefined members of the writing group, all will be co-authors as they fulfill the four authorship criteria:

_____
_____
_____
_____
_____

Additional persons who will be offered involvement in the manuscript process (authorship criteria two, three and four). Typically 1-2 per participating centre, but more people may be involved.

_____
_____
_____
_____
_____
_____
_____
_____
_____

All the above-mentioned names will appear on the final manuscript in the byline as authors, and all other persons involved in the research project will be mentioned in the Acknowledgements section as contributors.

In order to be listed in the byline as an author, the criteria for manuscript workflow should be fulfilled (see Appendix B). Anyone not fulfilling these workflow criteria will be removed as authors from the byline and mentioned in the Acknowledgements section as contributors.

Contract about deadlines

Another contract that you can make and that each author should sign as early as possible concerns the time frame for writing and revision of the manuscript before submission to a journal. The reason why this can be helpful is that a potential author can then not on purpose delay the process in the writing phase if you have this signed contract.

This contract will define exact deadlines for each co-author of when they have to respond with first and second revisions and when they have to give their final approval for submission. A typical deadline could be two weeks for each revision and one or two days for final approval. This means that if the co-authors does not get back to you within these deadlines, then he or she will no longer ba a co-author but in stead be mentioned in the acknowledgements section as a contributor in stead.

I can assure you that this helps because then they will answer back to you within this time frame that they have agreed upon. However, the key here is to make them sign this authorship contract up front before the study starts and then you have it in writing.

APPENDIX B

Manuscript workflow for multi-centre trials

- Before initiating the study, any authorship issues will be clarified in the authorship contract (see Appendix A).

- The manuscript may be prepared by a writing group typically consisting of 3-5 members or may be drafted by the first author and then undergo critical revision among the co-authors.

- The authors in the byline of the manuscript may include more people than those participating in the writing group and this is clearly defined in the authorship contract.

BEFORE FIRST DRAFT

- *2-3 weeks before* the first manuscript draft is ready, the author in charge of manuscript drafting should notify all co-authors by e-mail.

FIRST REVISION

- When distributing the manuscript draft to the co-authors, it should be pointed out that each co-author has e.g. a maximum of *two weeks* to revise the manuscript draft.

- If the co-author is not able to complete the revision within the timeframe, the author in charge of manuscript drafting should be notified as soon as possible.

- If a co-author does not report back in time, he/she should no longer be considered an author (cf. ICMJE authorship criterion two).

- After the specified timeframe, the author in charge of manuscript drafting prepares a new draft based on all co-authors' revisions.

SECOND REVISION

- Next, the author in charge of the manuscript distributes a new manuscript draft to the co-authors with clearly identifiable corrections, and each co-author has e.g. *one week* to revise the new manuscript draft.

- Again, if the co-author is unable to complete the revision in time, the author in charge of the manuscript should be notified as soon as possible.

FINAL APPROVAL

- When the manuscript is finished and ready for submission, it should be sent to all co-authors for final approval (ICMJE authorship criterion three). The co-authors should be given only e.g. *two days* to respond to the final approval of the manuscript. The final approval is given by e-mail as a response back to the author in charge of the manuscript and thereafter the manuscript can be submitted to a journal.

Revision of the manuscript after editorial response from a journal

- There are no strict rules regarding involvement of co-authors in the revision process, although it may be considered good ethical behavior to at least get critical revisions and a final approval from all co-authors before submitting the revised manuscript.

- Thus, most often the first and last author will collaborate on the preparation of a revised version of the manuscript taking into account all the issues raised by the editor and peer-reviewers. The final revised manuscript together with a cover letter describing all the changes made will then be sent to all co-authors for final approval before re-submission to the journal. A fair amount of time for this process of final approval would be e.g. *one week*.

- Final approval of the revised manuscript should be given as e-mail responses from the co-authors back to the author in charge of the manuscript before submission.

Signatures:
_____
_____
_____
_____
_____
_____
_____
_____

In small studies typically run in a single department, or if it a study inly involving your own research group then these authorship contracts may be overkill. However, if the study involves more than one department and especially if you work with people that you have not worked with previously, then is is advisable to make authorship contracts and have them signed before accrual of the first patient.

It is often practically impossible to involve all the contributors in the study as formal authors on the final manuscript. That is why you have to decide the criteria for authorship on your specific study before the study actually starts enrolling patients and the proposal here is to make two formal authorship contracts that can be found in the cited paper from Danish Medical Journal. Make all the participating departments sign these contracts and then you are ready to go.

Other contracts

All contracts should be in place before you start patient accrual. Besides the necessary permissions from the local ethics committee and other mandatory "official" contracts you will very often have to make formal agreements with other stakeholders in your organisation. This could for interventional pharmacological trials include the unit for good clinical practice, and it could include various research collaborators involved in your study. The research collaborators could be agreements with other laboratories, both in your own institution or in other hospitals or basic science institutions.

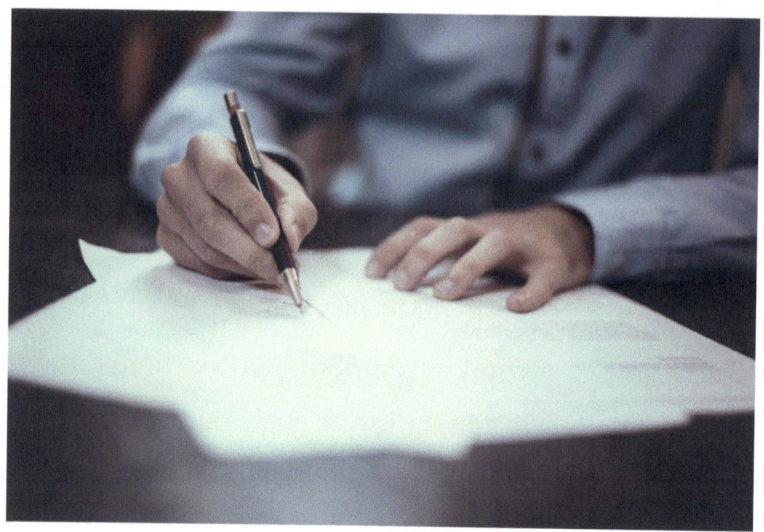

Although you may be good friends and have even worked together before, it could be a good idea to write down what you have actually agreed upon, meaning what analyses they will make, time frame and how much it will cost. It could also be relevant to make contracts with pathology departments or microbiologists depending on your study design.

Depending on the study it could be, especially for the larger interventional trials and especially when they are externally funded, be relevant to have formal contracts with an external CRO. Such a contract will need formal approval by your department head, and depending on your local organisation, often also by a legal department in the hospital or hospital system.

Permissions

Before you can start your accrual of patients or gathering of clinical data of any kind you have to get permissions from various places.

Ethics committee approval
Some of these permissions are "generic", meaning that it will be the same all over the World, and other permissions depend on what country you live in. For instance approval from an Ethics Committee is universal because all studies involving humans will have to follow the Helsinki Declaration and in this declaration it says explicitly that all human trials should be approved by an Ethics Committee before they can start.

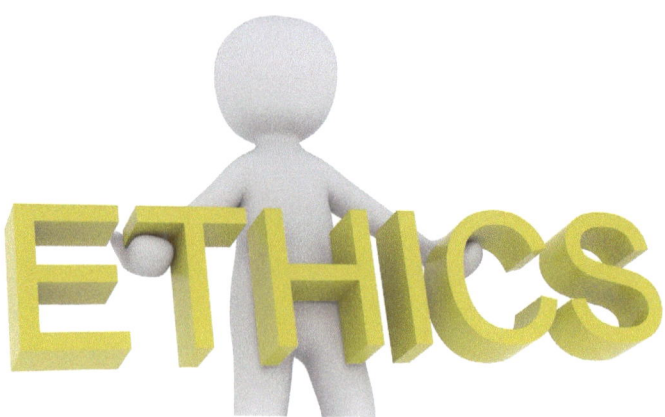

The exact local organisation is different in different countries. In some places it may be an institutional review board (an IRB) in a single hospital. Other countries may have committees covering a geographical region, and other countries may have a national system instead. All together, your study has to be approved by an ethics committee before you can start accruing patients.

Permission from local management
The next thing is generic too and that is the permission from your local management. If you are working in a clinical department you have to get approval from the head of the department, otherwise you cannot start your study. If you work in a research lab the same rules apply, you have to somehow get approval from your chief before you can start.

Data protection
The next point is different from country to country and that is the need for permission from a data protection agency (or similar). In the European Union there is an EU-directive regarding

protection of personal data and this directive has been approved by all the member countries. All countries have made their own laws based on this European Union directive (a EU directive is not a law). For instance in Denmark where I live there is an explicit law on data protection and therefore we have to get formal approval from The Danish Data Protection Agency every time we do research involving patients. These rules are actually quite strict but they can easily be fulfilled if you just do it correctly every time. In other countries it is more or less the same but of course it is called different things. Therefore, in Europe it is not a major problem because every member country has to follow their laws for personal data protection.

011100101110011101011
100011001010100101010
10101101101011011011
11101011HACKED11110110
000101010010001011111
100101010101010101010100
111110011111011001000

In the United States it is a little different because the US has not a formal centralised legislation at the federal level regarding this issue. However, the US does ensure privacy and protection of data through the United States Privacy Act, The Safe Harbor Act and The Health Insurance Portability and Accountability Act. This means that the patient may be secured in a similar fashion as in the European Union, but it is just handled a little bit differently. In the US if you are running an NIH-sponsored phase-3 clinical trial, then you are required to have a data and safety monitoring board. This will consist of a group of experts that will oversee your research study so that the patients will not be in danger. Also you have to get permission from the FDA (Food and Drug Administration) for these large clinical trials before you can start.

Different study types - different rules
There may be local differences about required permissions fro different study types. In my country (Denmark), we do not need permission from the ethics committee if we do a study only

with questionnaires without biological material. The same applies for focus group interviews and database studies. In all studies, however, we need permission from the Data Protection Agency because we are registering personal data.

If we do a prospective study where we gather data from patients prospectively even though it is not invasive, then we need to have approval from The Ethics Committee, and again also of course from the Data protection Agency.

If it is something that we could call quality assurance research, meaning that we want to see e.g. how it went with a certain type of surgical procedure then we do not need ethics committee approval but only permission from the Data Protection Agency.

If we are testing drugs or devices then it is of course very much different. Now we need approvals from the ethics committee, the Data Protection Agency, the Health Authorities (in Denmark it is called the National Board of Health and that corresponds to the FDA in the US), the Unit for Good Clinical Practice, and the Data Protection Agency.

You always have to follow the local laws and

regulations. The means for a multinational study, that every country or study site have to follow their local rules and regulations.

Registrations

If you do a clinical trial, then you have to register your study in a publicly available database such as www.clinicaltrials.gov. This database is a good choice for your registration because it is free of charge and quite easy to operate. If you do not register the trial before accrual of the first patient then it will be very difficult to get it published. Almost all journals adhere to these guidelines from the International Committee of Medical Journal Editors (www.icmje.org).

It is not mandatory to register an observational study, but many studies in www.clinicaltrials.gov are in fact observational studies. So why not register these as well. Registration will increase transparency and will be regarded as positive by the journal editor and peer reviewers.

It is not mandatory to register a systematic review, but it is highly recommended. A systematic review can be registered in the PROSPERO database which is situated in the UK and it is free of charge.

Clinicaltrials.gov

As you may recall the ICMJE made it mandatory to register clinical trials before the trial was initiated. This means that the trial has to be registered in a public database before the inclusion of the first patient in the trial. This led to a large increase in the number of registered trials in for instance clinicaltrials.gov which is the largest trial registry available.

Clinicaltrials.gov is financed by the American taxpayers and we are grateful to our American friends that they will pay for this. If you look at the trials registered in clinicaltrials.gov it is astonishing that less than half of the studies actually comes from the US. As of today (March 2018), the number of trials registered is 269,000 and the number of trials from the US is only 110,000. You can see the geographical distribution at this web-address: https://clinicaltrials.gov/ct2/search/map.

So if you wonder where to register your trial, I will say why not use the biggest one: clinicaltrials.gov. The demand from the ICMJE was that trials should be registered in a publicly available and searchable trial registry and for some reason (and honestly I do not understand why) – there are more than 20 different trial registries around the World. Many countries have decided to make their own registries, but why ? Why not just use the American which is free of charge and with very good functionality.

Search across registries
It would be a lot easier if all trials were registered in the same registry. If you want to find a trial you can of course go to clinicaltrials.gov and search for the trial but this does not cover all trips around the globe. The easiest way to find a trial will actually be to go somewhere else. WHO has made an international clinical trial registry platform search portal which is again quite easi to use. The web-address is http://apps.who.int/trialsearch/

This search portal will collect data from different registries and they get data once a week from the Australian New Zealand Clinical Trials Registry, the Chinese Clinical Trial Registry, clinicaltrials.gov, from EU Clinical Trials Register, ISRCTN, and from the Netherlands National Trial Register. Every four weeks they collect data from the Brazilian Clinical Trials Registry (ReBec), the Clinical Trials Registry - India, the Clinical Research Information Service - Republic of Korea, the Cuban Public Registry of Clinical Trials, the German Clinical Trials Register, the Iranian Registry of Clinical Trials, the Japan Primary Registries Network, the Pan African Clinical Trial Registry, the Sri Lanka Clinical Trials Registry, the Thai Clinical Trials Register (TCTR), and the Peruvian Clinical Trials Registry (REPEC).

All these different registries provide data for the WHO search portal so if you don't need to be absolutely updated with your search - because some of the data may be up to 4 weeks old - you can go to the WHO portal and then make your search.

Which trials should be registered
The demand from ICMJE was that clinical trials have to be registered. So what is a clinical trial? A clinical trial is in this context defined as an interventional study, meaning that you are testing an effect of some kind of intervention in humans. This also means that animal studies are not covered and observational studies were not

originally meant to be included. However, as mentioned above, many registered studies are in fact observational in their design.

If I should look at this from the editor's point of view I would say that there is no reason not to support this development because the original thought about trial registration was to make it transparent and to ensure that all trials that are initiated in patients will actually somehow be publicly available. Furthermore, the registration should ensure that the original study design should be valid all the way to publication, i.e. The authors should not be able to change primary outcome or make other "tricks" to get a better result than originally possible with their study design. In other words the authors should not go on fishing expeditions in their results after the study is completed.

Conclusion

If you have an interventional or observational study the go for trial registration and I will personally recommend clinicaltrials.gov because it is free of charge with good functionality and it is the largest of the approved registries.

There is also a possibility to register systematic reviews or meta-analyses. This is not mandatory at the moment, but you have the possibility to register those studies at the PROSPERO database. This is hosted by University of York (UK) and you can google PROSPERO and University of York and then you get the link for this register. This will also give a registration number that you can put in your scientific paper.

Reporting guidelines

In recent years it has become much more common to use a reporting guideline when writing a scientific paper. The purpose of using a guideline for reporting your results in a scientific paper is primarily to increase the quality of the research. It will also make it easier for the reader because different papers will be written in more or less the same way and therefore it will be easier to understand the design, the execution and the analyses of the studies. Thus, there are very good reasons to use a reporting guidelines when writing your paper.

Another good reason to use a reporting guideline is that it will in many cases increase your change of getting your paper accepted for publication by a journal and the reason for that is that the journal editors also like very much these guidelines because they will make the papers better. Often the use of a reporting guideline will heighten the quality of the research papers so use a reporting guideline if at all possible.

Equator Network

You can find all the different guidelines in one single place on the Internet at equator-network.org. Here you can find links to all available guidelines, and there are many I can assure you. Right now (March 2018) there are 398 available guidelines and you can find links to all these on the equator network homepage.

The guidelines are divided in specific guidelines and generic guidelines. If you can use a generic guideline then do it because it will increase your chance of getting your paper accepted for publication. There are links to the guideline itself, typically also a check-list, maybe a flow-diagram, templates etc. So go to the equator network homepage and find your guideline and then follow that.

Some examples of generic guidelines are for instance the CONSORT guideline for randomised clinical trials, the PRISMA guideline for systematic reviews and meta-analyses, the STROBE guideline for observational studies, the CARE guideline for case reports, and the COREQ guideline for interview studies and focus group interviews. There are links on the equator network homepage to all these different guidelines. The individual linked webpages are typically called by the acronym and statement, e.g. consort-statement.org or prisma-statement.org and you can find links on the equator network home page.

The generic guidelines are most often known by the editors whereas the specific guidelines are more rare and not very often known by the editors actually. So use a generic guideline if possible. It will increase the quality of your research and also provide transparency of the research process. Therefore, it is a very good idea to go to equator network and get your guideline.

Chapter 4:
Last minute preparations

Practical data management

There are important practical issues about data management meaning where to store the trial data both during as well as after the trial.

Electronic data

It is of course tempting to use <u>web-based solutions</u> like Dropbox or OneDrive or whatever they are called out there but this is not OK. The reason is that you cannot be sure that the identity of the patients is protected and therefor it is not allowed - not even if you pseudo-anonymise the data.

Then what about your personal working <u>computer in your office</u>? Can you put your trial data there? The answer is again unfortunately no, because this computer may be stolen, so you cannot be sure that the information will not end in the wrong hands.

You can use <u>encrypted USB</u> memory sticks. That is actually an OK solution, but they have to be encrypted with an access code and you have to of course keep those USB-sticks behind locked doors. In my country we have to keep them behind two locked doors. I am honestly not sure that it will help with two doors in stead of one, but these are the rules. There has to be two locks for a thief to go through in order to steel those USB sticks. You can buy commercially encrypted USB sticks. They are a little more expensive than conventional USB sticks, but it is not a fortune. So it is actually a good solution to use.

Another thing that you can do is to put your data on a <u>network drive</u> in your office, in your hospital or where you work, but this network drive has to be a closed drive meaning that only you have access to that special drive or place on the network server. You will have contact your IT-specialist in order to set this up. This is also a good solution because the network will be backed regularly so your data will be safe.

Data on paper

When we are talking about the paper versions of the CRFs then they also have to be kept in a place where nobody can get to them other then if these persons are part of the study. So, like the encrypted USB sticks, these paper version CRFs have to be locked away. - in my country behind two locked doors but there may be other routines in your country. Thus, you have to check it and of course follow these rules.

After the study

When the study is finished and you have to save the paper version of the CRFs as well as the electronic files such as electronic CRFs, Excel files, or statistical software files. All these things have to be saved in exactly the same manor as during your study and this means behind a locked door solution of some kind and then for a number of years according to your local regulations.

Why run a mock patient?

Before starting the actual patient accrual for your scientific project it is a very good idea to run a mock patient. This means that you simulate a real patient and thereby will go through all the different phases of the practical running of the study with a simulated patient. It could be a research colleague or even a real patient, but without performing the intended trial interventions.

The reason why it is a good idea to run a mock patient is that you will discover many practical details that need to be refined before you start your actual patient accrual. It could be small things like having the correct tubes for blood sampling, the correct labels or to give you a realistic estimate of the necessary time that you need to spend on every patient and every detailed phase of the trial.

This may be vital information in the practical management of your research study and thereby it is highly recommended to run a mock patient before you start your actual patient accrual. It may cost you a day's work, but it is well spent.

Who is going to help you?

In the planning of your study it is very important to be realistic about the practical work that will be necessary for patient accrual and data sampling. You really need to discuss this in detail with your mentor in order to plan things realistically. If you try to run a clinical trial and do not have established the necessary work force, then it can be very stressful and ultimately result in the study not being completed as planned.

There is no need to be a hero when planning a clinical trial. The important thing is that the trial will be finished on time and without any casualties (you!).

Typical helpers could be research colleagues, medical students or research nurses. There are many possibilities and it is advisable to consider this practical clinical planning point in detail before you start your research trial.

Last minute activity

Now you are almost ready to include the first patient in your clinical trial. You have considered all the practical issues in your research project and have prepared according to rules and regulations. Everything should be in place now and it is time to make the absolutely final preparations before the first patient is included.

These final preparations will include checking your trial master file to see if all permissions and forms are in place. You will check the case report forms and ensure that you have one case report form for each patient and that this form will include all necessary papers to obtain the planned variables for each patient.

Depending on the project design it could be a good idea to make a small basket for each patient with the necessary equipment, papers, a pen, etc. Whatever is needed for the first patient. Then you can take this patient's specific basket in your hand and approach the first patient.

Before the actual first patient, it is important that you have obtained all the necessary permissions for various regulatory authorities but also, and very important, from the head of department and all the other key persons that need to support you indirectly. Do not forget to talk to the local leaders and get their backing.

Chapter 5:
Closing

Closing remarks

Congratulations! You have now made it to the end of this book and hopefully you have learned some important lessons about study planning before you get to inclusion of the first patient in your clinical trial.

There are many issues to consider in this preparation phase and perhaps most importantly you will have to get a mentor where you enjoy your collaboration. I will also strongly advise you to start the research process by producing a systematic review within the field of your research question.

There are many rules and regulations that you have to comply with along the way and you will find the answers to most of these questions in the text in this book. You will also have to discuss it in detail with your scientific mentor because it is of course important not to make a short-cut in the planning phase and all rules have to be followed.

However, don't be depressed about all the rules and regulations because it is actually not so difficult when you just follow the rules for registrations and obtaining permissions. If you do not get all the necessary permissions, then you will have serious problems later on when you want to get your paper published in in some countries there will also be personal legal consequences for you. That is why there is no escape from this area, so you might as well follow the rules without any exceptions.

If it is possible for you in your research environment to run a mock patient befor the actual patient inclusion I would strongly recommend that. This will show you where you have weak spots and it will make life much easier when the real study is running.

I hope that I have explained the study planning phases for you so that you will be better prepared when you will include your first patient in your clinical trial. I know that there are many issues to consider in the planning phase, but do not despair because it is actually not so difficult. The main purpose of the preparation phase is besides getting the necessary permissions also, or actually most importantly, to increase the quality of your research project. Good preparation will ensure good data quality and that will in turn help getting your paper published in a good biomedical journal.

Other books in this series

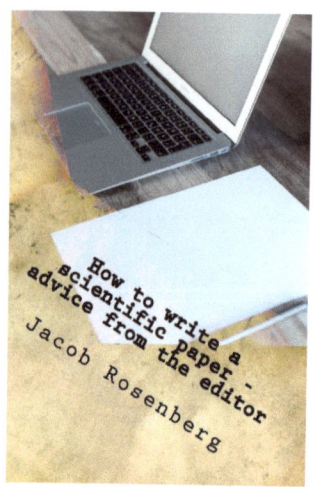

How to write a scientific paper: advice from the editor. Ultimate Researcher's Guide Series, Volume 1.

Available as paperback and kindle edition on all Amazon platforms.

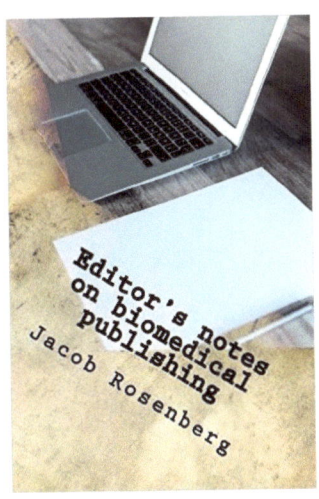

Editor's notes on biomedical publishing. Ultimate Researcher's Guide Series, Volume 2.

Available as paperback and kindle edition on all Amazon platforms.

About the author

Jacob Rosenberg (1964) was born and grew up in Copenhagen, Denmark. He is professor of surgery at the University of Copenhagen, and chief surgeon at the Gastro-unit, surgical section, Herlev Hospital (also in Copenhagen).

The author page at amazon.com is: https://www.amazon.com/author/jacobrosenberg

Notes

Notes

Contact information

jacob.rosenberg@regionh.dk

www.ingramcontent.com/pod-product-compliance
Lightning Source LLC
Chambersburg PA
CBHW041940240526
45473CB00033B/13